WEAR AND TEAR

STOP THE PAIN AND PUT THE SPRING BACK IN YOUR BODY

DR. BOB ARNOT

SIMON & SCHUSTER
New York London Toronto Sydney

SIMON & SCHUSTER
Rockefeller Center
1230 Avenue of the Americas
New York, NY 10020

First Simon & Schuster trade paperback edition 2004

SIMON & SCHUSTER and colophon are registered trademarks
of Simon & Schuster, Inc.

For information about special discounts for bulk purchases,
please contact Simon & Schuster Special Sales at
1-800-456-6798 or business@simonandschuster.com.

Designed by Rhea Braunstein
Illustrations by Alexis Seabrook

Manufactured in the United States of America

1 3 5 7 9 10 8 6 4 2

The Library of Congress has cataloged the hardcover edition as follows:

Arnot, Robert Burns.
Wear and tear : stop the pain and put the spring back
in your body / Bob Arnot.
p. cm.
Includes bibliographical references and index.
1. Osteoarthritis—Prevention. 2. Physical fitness. 3. Health.
I. Title.
RC931.O67 A334 2003
616.7'223—dc21   2002030871

ISBN 0-7432-2555-4
0-7432-2556-2 (Pbk)

This publication contains the opinions and ideas of its author. It is intended to provide helpful and informative material on the subjects addressed in the publication. It is sold with the understanding that the author and publisher are not engaged in rendering medical, health, or any other kind of personal professional services in the book. The reader should consult his or her medical, health, or other competent professional before adopting any of the suggestions in this book or drawing inferences from it.

The author and publisher specifically disclaim all responsibility for any liability, loss, or risk, personal or otherwise, which is incurred as a consequence, directly or indirectly, of the use and application of any of the contents of this book.

*This book is dedicated to
Carrie Arnot*

ACKNOWLEDGMENTS

Geoff Kloske: Geoff was the perfect editor, incisive and skillful. He always had fresh and inspiring ideas on how to make this book even better. I'll always be grateful to Geoff for the compassion he showed when my father died suddenly during this project. I'll never forget his understanding and help.

David Rosenthal: Special thanks to David Rosenthal, my publisher, for having the vision to make *Wear and Tear* happen and for putting such an outstanding team behind it. I prize David for his unending enthusiasm and great good nature, which were sources of wonderful inspiration.

Suzanne C. Bagin: My associate in writing this book, Suzanne showed ceaseless energy and amazing attention to detail. Her inquisitive mind and investigative skills brought a treasure trove of wonderful material to this book. Her ability to work tirelessly while I was abroad, reporting on the war against terror, kept this book on track and on schedule.

Dan and Simon Green: To my indefatigable agents who've always been there for me, for their hard work and devotion.

CONTENTS

CONTENTS

INTRODUCTION: WEAR AND TEAR

One day it hit me hard. I was stunned by the things I could no longer do. I couldn't squat and come back up without putting my hand on a chair. I couldn't walk a mile without excruciating, deep-seated, aching right hip pain. I couldn't bend over to play with my six-year-old son. It was hard getting out of a chair. My hips seemed to freeze after a brief hike. Calisthenics had become a cruel ritual, like a spymaster's exquisite torture.

They call it wear and tear. After decades of iron-man contests, ski racing, cross-country ski racing, kayaking, rowing, running, swimming, mountain climbing, you name it, I was worn and torn. Ugh! Too bad, you may say, but I'm not alone! From couch potatoes to weekend warriors, we're getting worn to the bone years earlier than our parents.

I have good company, and lots of it. Days before the beginning of the Olympic Games in Sydney, Australia, more than a dozen NBC Sports commentators were groaning and creaking on treadmills, stair machines, exercise bikes, and weight-training gear in the health club on the top floor of the Inter-Continental Hotel. Most were in their late twenties or early thirties. These ex-Olympians turned broadcasters put in the time to stay their best, but now they all suffered from the aches and pains of wear and tear. The swimmers complained about bad backs, the gymnasts about their wrists, the divers their necks, the wrestlers their knees. Wear and tear was showing up in these athletes well before age forty.

We're all getting worn and torn faster and younger than ever before. Why? We're putting more and more of the wrong kind of strain on our joints at earlier and earlier ages. Some of us overload our joints by being overweight. Others because we're too active in all the wrong sports. For many, it's just plain walking the wrong way. "Disuse, misuse, and abuse" is fast becoming the slogan of our generation. The fact is, we're all getting visibly worn and torn in bits and pieces starting in our thirties, though for some of us the process may begin in our teens. By age forty, wear and tear already shows up on our X rays!

At this point you may say, Hey, come on, Dr. Bob, more bad news? Well, there's lots of good news. I won't spoil the story for you, but in my own remarkable journey, I'm happy to report that you can beat wear and tear and become more supple, limber, flexible, and energetic than ever before and the pain will be *gone!* The earlier you start the better, but whatever stage you're at, *Wear and Tear* has the answers. Remember, for most of us wear and tear *is* aging. Wear and tear saps the most important elements of our youth leaving in its place creaky, groaning joints; tired, sore, inflexible muscles. I'm a little reluctant to mention the "A" word—arthritis—but that's where excessive wear and tear eventually leads. For most, this book will help you detect the early warning signs of wear and tear before arthritis rears its ugly head, so you can delay or prevent it entirely. The concept of prevention in arthritis is so new, the gift wrapping is still barely off the package, but there's lots you can do—from identifying a faulty gait and cushioning the blows to your joints to rescuing damaged cartilage. For those of you who already have the beginnings of arthritis, this book will give you the realistic advice for beating it. For those of you with more serious arthritis, there's great hope that you can beat the pain and disability you now suffer. Chances are that if you already suffer from muscle and joint aches and pains after activity, you're already on the way to wear-and-tear arthritis.

WEAR AND TEAR, A UNIQUE KIND OF ARTHRITIS: OSTEOARTHRITIS

Throughout this book, when the word "arthritis" is used, it refers only to wear-and-tear arthritis, also known as osteoarthritis, nicknamed "OA." What's the difference between wear and tear and arthritis? Wear and tear is pure mechanical damage. Arthritis occurs when this mechanical damage triggers chemical reactions within a joint that causes its destruction. The British have separate terms for them. They call the mechanical destruction of joints by wear and tear "arthrosis" and its chemical transformation "arthritis." Eric L. Radin, M.D., professor emeritus of orthopedic surgery at Tufts University School of Medicine, emphasizes the difference: "Arthritis is a joint problem primarily from metabolic or inflammatory causes; arthrosis is a joint problem initially from mechanical abnormalities."

I didn't honestly make much of my own aches and pains until I was asked to moderate a panel discussion at an arthritis meeting. Maybe it was denial, or maybe I just didn't put the whole picture together the way I would have if I had been examining a patient. I walked into the lecture room to greet the panelists. A very sweet young woman from the Arthritis Foundation came up to me. "Gee, you've got a limp! Do you have arthritis?" she asked with glee, perhaps sizing me up as a new poster boy for the illness. Not the rheumatoid type she meant, but plain old wear-and-tear arthritis. Had I become one of "them"? Was I an arthritic? Of course not, I protested. I tried to escape the watchful eye of Joe Montana, the panel's special guest and former 49ers quarterback. A little arthritis, Bob, he asked? No, no, no, I protested again. I don't have arthritis. But Joe's unwavering look and practiced eye sure gave me second thoughts! I considered it over the weekend and then called a terrific orthopedic surgeon in New York first thing Monday morning. I described my symptoms. He suggested an appointment. After I reported to the hospital and stripped down to my shorts, he examined my knee, while a small group looked on. "Overloaded," he said. Then he looked at my hip. He maneuvered it until there was a distinct clash of bone on bone. Ouch! He said, "You probably don't want to know what this is!" I said I did. He hustled me off to the X-ray room. After a brief wait, he called me back in to look at the X ray. Sure enough, the film showed a joint already badly damaged. He advised me to give up skiing, tennis, and running. I was given a series of modest exercises to do and sent packing. Nothing seemed to help. Traditional medicine would have nothing to offer until I was ready for a joint replacement: no effective therapy, no medications, and no exercises to repair my damaged hip. I swore to myself: "I'll be back, better than ever!" Not as an Olympian or Super Bowl champ but as the ultimate weekend warrior of my youth. I hired an assistant and began to comb the scientific literature. I read every article in every journal. I visited the best labs and clinics in the country. I put together my own program with the help of dozens of top specialists and everything I learned is in this book.

Now I've beaten wear and tear, and you can too. I feel and perform better than at any time since my twenties. I have a new outlook on life. I'd like to share my quest with you in the hope that you can prevent wear and tear if it hasn't yet struck, or intervene and stop it in its tracks if it has. Within weeks of the arthritis meeting, I went from taking twelve Advils a day to none. I went from having to stumble down the aisle of a commuter airline to walking pain-free. I found I could play singles tennis again without the cruel dark ache I'd suffered from before. The leg spasms that kept me awake at night are gone. I can jump off a precipice into the steepest couloir in Jackson Hole, surf the toughest onshore break at Bondi Beach, Australia—all the things I wanted to do as a kid but never dared! In one of my earlier books, *Turning Back the Clock,* I wrote about reversing many of the effects of aging. Since then I've learned that no effects of aging are more important to stave off than those affecting your muscles and joints. Why? Muscles and joints bear the major brunt of wear and tear. As muscles become stiff and joints become sore and restricted in their range of motion, you begin to actually look older and feel older. The secrets you'll learn in this book will help you recover that lost youth by putting spring back in your step and adding dramatic increases in agility and flexibility. You can use this book for solving individual problems on an à la carte basis or follow the whole program. You may say ugh! Who wants to get involved in a long, drawn out program! The great good news is how *fast* you'll feel better—in weeks, not months or years. I've also tried to be realistic, making the steps easily manageable during a busy workday.

I've called this book *Wear and Tear* because it's a whole lot less depressing than mentioning the "A" word, arthritis! Also, wear and tear doesn't affect just the joints; it begins with worn-out, stiff muscles, tendons, ligaments, and bones. Arthritis is the final culmination of a long process of wear and tear, a process you can slow, stop, or even reverse—if you act now! You will have a decades-long betrothal with arthritis before you are married to the disease. But those decades contain years of aches and pains, stiffness, and loss of function before the searing pain brings the disease home. X rays show that by midlife, 50 percent of us will be affected.* In the weight-bearing joints, particularly the hip and knee, this degeneration accelerates with age. By the seventh decade, it affects an astounding 85 percent of us.

Every single person I talk to has some wear and tear. I mean honestly from my thirteen-year-old son to twenty-year-old snowboarders, thirty-year-old skiers, forty-year-old tennis players, fifty-year-old runners, right up to my eighty-seven-year-old parents. It amazes me that my parents developed the aches and pains in their eighties that we are developing in our forties. Times have changed! The paradoxical pairing of frantic overactivity at one end of the spectrum and overindulgent, underactive lifestyles at the other end is ripping us apart years earlier. How widespread is wear and tear?

---

* D. T. Felson, "The Epidemiology of Knee Osteoarthritis: Results from the Framingham Osteoarthritis Study," *Seminars in Arthritis Rheumatology* 20 (1990): 42–50.

I've been unable to have a conversation with *anyone* who isn't suffering from it. For instance, riding the fire-engine-red gondola up Mount Mansfield, my local ski area, I sat with a father and son. The father, age sixty-three, had a torn rotator cuff and a torn meniscus for which he was taking a supplement called glucosamine. The thirty-two-year-old son already had torn cartilage in his hip from an aggressive snowboarding stance and had the pain to prove it.

This book's great news is that if you're like me, you suffer from a whole host of rapidly reversible conditions, the most significant of which I call "stiff man syndrome." Many are the consequence of how we live, the most interesting of which are practices of daily living abandoned by many Americans but still practiced by millions of people in China, India, and Africa—millions who never develop wear and tear.

THE ROAD MAP

This book will give you a unique and exceptionally useful set of tools to beat wear and tear.

From the earliest stages of wear and tear to the most severe, I'll take you through powerful and highly targeted steps. I'll also give you my own consumer experience—what really worked for me and what was no more than hype! For those of you pressed for time, there are a half-dozen deceptively simple yet elegant steps, taking fifteen minutes a day, that will rapidly relieve your pain and renew your muscles, tendons, and joints. If you're a full-on weekend warrior, there's a lot more! Many chapters have self-tests to determine what your individual needs are. You'll find that most of the solutions offered are "off the shelf." That makes them inexpensive and easily available. Since the more measures you take, the better protected you will be, you'll find it easy, in many cases, to treat yourself. I've searched the globe to find *the* most effective steps there are. The book is divided into two parts. Part One clearly presents major problems you may have that accelerate wear and tear. Part Two contains the best, most innovative and exciting solutions to these problems.

The book employs the principles of evidence-based medicine as proposed by McMaster University: "the health care provider must use his/her clinical judgment based on the evidence as well as incorporating his/her values and the patients' values with regard to the types of treatments that they want to take as well as the degree of risk they are willing to entail." For that reason you won't find a single recipe but rather personal choices customized to address your specific results on a series of these simple tests and the amount of time and effort you want to put into beating wear and tear. You may, for example, choose to pursue only two or three of the suggested solutions, yet you will find that even these make a major improvement in your ability to beat wear and tear. These may be completely passive steps that take no effort or, if you're trying to restore your athletic career, you may want to undertake more aggressive steps.

Here's the road map for beating wear and tear:

PART ONE: PROBLEMS—WHAT CAUSES WEAR AND TEAR

The conventional wisdom holds that wear and tear is a dumb disease. You're older, live with it! Like an old set of springs on a pickup truck, one day your joints are going to go. Wear and tear used to be a dull backwater of modern medicine, but now elegant scientific research has uncovered a fresh way of understanding wear and tear. The big concept is that wear and tear is a biomechanical disease, meaning that faulty movement patterns and mechanical flaws in our skeletal alignments create a force that, over time, tears our muscles, ligaments, and joints apart. These are called "movement performance problems." These mechanical forces then lead to biochemical changes in the joint and its ultimate destruction. For each problem chapter in Part One, there is a matching solution chapter in Part Two. Part One will help you assess your own needs with a series of simple self-tests. In Part Two you'll be able to choose solutions for yourself based on those needs.

What are those mechanical forces? Here's a brief look.

Heel Pounders

Are you a microklutz? That's the term Oxford University researchers use for those of us who pound our heels on the ground as we walk. If you add to that poor muscular power and coordination, you may pound your joints with forces greater than your body weight. Oxford researchers found that a sharp heel strike alone predicted early, prearthritic knee pain in young people. Imagine discovering that in your twenties! You'd prevent a lifetime of knee pain. This pounding stiffens the bone underlying the cartilage. As that bone becomes harder and harder, it begins to pulverize the cartilage, slowly destroying it over time. It's amazing to think that just plain *walking* could destroy your joints! In fact, this may be the biggest single insight that researchers have had: it's not the occasional game of tennis that does your joints in—it's walking! Why? Repetitive forces are generated by tens of thousands of steps a day. So struck are some researchers that they recommend *against* walking as a form of exercise for people with certain "fatal flaws." If you're a person who walks across a floor and gets everyone's attention just by the intensity of your heel strike, you've got a problem! You're a "ripper," short for someone with an extreme degree of repetitive impulse loading. Rippers have hard-and-fast joint loading without adequate shock absorption. This repetitive impulse loading is found before X-ray changes. Combine that with the "fatal flaws" found in Chapter 3, such as high-arched feet or bowleggedness, and you'll be arthritic far sooner than you should be!

Proper biomechanics applies to how you sit, push, pull, bend, and walk. What's the one activity that could grind away joints day in and day out?

Again, it's walking! In fact, research shows that an improper landing while walking can load your knee joint with an instantaneous force per second eighty-four times greater than your body weight. Do that day in, day out, and there's little wonder that you'd suffer wear and tear and eventually arthritis! What can you do? Blunt the impact. Proper shoes, heel inserts, and learning how to walk more gently will all do the trick. Learning how to walk "on air" can protect your joints and eliminate your pain. We'll look at some fun, innovative ways to improve your gait to kill your pain.

Stiff Man Syndrome

The indulgences of modern living have hit us hardest around the waistline. However, our lifestyle is also hitting us where it hurts most: in our joints. Through lack of use, our tendons and muscles shorten and tighten. As they do, they change the mechanics of how joints work, helping to slowly destroy them. Chapter 2 takes a fascinating look at other cultures that get very little wear and tear despite having a longer life expectancy than Americans. These are cultures, for example, in which people still squat rather than sit on chairs, and they maintain full use of their hips and knees. You'll read how tendons are re-formed as shorter, thicker, less elastic, and far less mobile. Some simple tests will help you determine what range of motion your limbs should have. The companion chapter in Part Two is "Restore Your Joints."

Fatal Flaws

Human joints should last a lifetime, even a very long one. Why do some of our joints wear out faster? Simply put, flaws in our skeletal system create imbalances, like a worn out bearing in a car's transmission. Skeletal malalignment can alter how weight is distributed across the joint surface. Over many years that unbalanced pressure on the cartilage can lead to early and severe wear-and-tear arthritis. I call these "fatal flaws."

We'll look at simple ways to detect the most common fatal flaws such as bowlegs and knock knees so you can take steps to balance the pressure across your joints. For instance, a high-tech knee brace can instantly redistribute the load across your knee. With simple self-tests, you'll be able to determine if you may have a ticking time bomb in your skeleton.

The most important fatal flaws may not be the ones you're born with. Orthopedic surgeons are becoming increasingly concerned about the small injuries we suffer over the years. These are called "subclinical" traumas because we often suffer little pain or disability at the time and may not even visit the doctor. However, these minor injuries can create microfractures in our joint surfaces. Over time, doctors worry that the daily pounding our joints receive hammers on these weak points until the cartilage becomes worn and arthritis begins. The solution is identifying these early injuries and the associated weakness. Teens who suffer knee injuries are at greatly increased risk of wear-and-tear arthritis. The sports boom of the sixties, seventies, and eighties is turning into the arthritis boom of the twenty-first century. And it's not just sports; if your occupation requires you to kneel or squat for long periods of time, you're also at significantly increased risk of arthritis. The companion chapter in Part Two is "Fix the Flaws."

The Weak Link

Subtle losses of muscular leg strength put you at high risk for early wear and tear. Weak muscles lead to unstable joints. During activity, that instability results in excessive movement of the joint. What's worse, the muscles around the joint can't react to awkward movements to protect the joint. This causes rapid, jarring loading of the joint that then damages the cartilage. In fact, weakness of the thigh muscle is one of the most common and early predictors of arthritis. It's a much better early warning sign than pain and appears well in advance of X-ray changes. At-home tests will help you determine if a simple lack of strength could send you down the path of getting worn and torn years earlier than you otherwise would. Many of us have almost imperceptible weakness from an innocuous injury. We think we've recovered and never give the injury a second thought, but the muscle is still weak and we slowly end up destroying our joints. The companion chapter in Part Two is "Build Protective Strength."

Overload

Excess body fat may lead to heart disease, diabetes, and a variety of other chronic illnesses. One of those diseases is early wear and tear. You'll be able to quickly determine if extra pounds are killing your joints. The companion chapter in Part Two is "Lighten the Load."

PART TWO: SOLUTIONS—BEATING WEAR AND TEAR

You'll find that the first chapters contain easy, simple, quick steps. These easy first steps will get you quickly on your way to beating wear and tear. They'll give you the confidence that the measures in this book are highly effective and motivate you to progress through the more strenuous efforts in the last part of Part Two. If you go no further, the first three steps are passive, requiring no physical effort yet effective enough to make a big difference.

Kill the Pain

Mick Jagger sang about a "mother's little helper." Many baby boomers' little helper is a brownish pill with a sweet candy taste called Advil. For aches and pains, there's nothing that works faster or better for me than its main ingredient, ibuprofen. But watch out! There's a multibillion-dollar industry backed by the full punch of a megamillion-dollar advertising budget, all targeted at your poor aching joints. But in the blizzard of information, the consumer is often left without the rules of engagement. Simply put, few of us know how to use the drug effectively. In this section we'll look at what works best and how to use it. I've surveyed the top practitioners in the field, who've shared the secrets they've learned over decades of practice.

From pain relief for sore muscles after the local 10-K run or club tennis match to treatment for wear-and-tear arthritis, this section has the most up-to-date treatment. For instance, did you know that many doctors are concerned that some analgesics might *worsen* arthritis? The fear is that they will mask the pain and you will do even more damage to your joints. One study actually shows much greater impact on the knee joint during walking in a patient with arthritis after a pain reliever has been taken. Even more troubling is the theory that pain relievers might inhibit joint repair through a process known as "analgesic arthropathy."

Pain relievers such as nonsteroidal anti-inflammatory drugs (NSAIDs), including Motrin and Advil, can blunt the repair capacity of specialized cells in the cartilage called chondrocytes. The good news is that there are medications that ease your pain and may also protect your joints. This is a thorough consumer's look at what works and what doesn't, including the new COX-2 inhibitors and topical creams, which treat your pain but may spare your stomach.

Protect Your Joints

Physical injury, hard heel strike, or other trauma is only the beginning of joint damage. These physical forces are translated into biochemical changes in the joint that ultimately destroy it. How? Mechanical forces trigger a biochemical chain reaction, resulting in a toxic soup. Your cartilage bathes in that toxic soup, which accelerates the damage to your joints and leads to further loss of cartilage as the joint surface weakens and softens. The main culprits are substances called "cytokines," which orchestrate the breakdown of the basic building blocks of cartilage.

Wear-and-tear arthritis may be the only disease in modern medicine where supplements are more powerful, more helpful, and safer than the available prescription drugs. Some top orthopedic surgeons at top medical centers such as the Hospital for Special Surgery would rather see their patients on supplements such as glucosamine than traditional pain relievers. Why? They're effective pain relievers that may not increase the risk of bleeding stomach ulcers as traditional drugs such as ibuprofen and aspirin can. There's also the advantage that, unlike analgesics, they may treat the underlying disease, beefing up thinning cartilage. In fact, the latest review in the journal *Lancet* shows that glucosamine may really protect the cartilage and slow down the disease! Glucosamine may interrupt this biochemical chain reaction by diluting the toxic soup of chemicals that bathes our joints.

We'll look at other sophisticated drugs already available in Europe and now clearing clinical trials and regulatory hurdles in America. Researchers believe that improving the way your joints work through physical training could make these drugs work even better.

Fix the Flaws

The wrong shoes increase the forces on your joints, compressing the knee by 23 percent more than normal. Imagine what good shoes can do! Shock-absorbing footwear and other devices can neutralize fatal flaws and dramatically reduce the mechanical forces that create wear and tear. For instance, we'll look at bubble-soled walking shoes with a soft arch and deformable heel for daily footwear. There's a complete guide to the best shoes to save your joints, plus other mechanical devices such as knee braces.

Restore Your Joints

The conventional wisdom holds that we stretch to loosen tight muscles. While that is certainly an enviable goal, it doesn't go nearly far enough. Over time, the natural range of motion of our joints shrinks dramatically. A consistent finding in patients with arthritis of the knee is decreased range of motion of the hip and ankle, as well as the knee. In this chapter you'll find how to increase the range of motion in all three joints by a remarkable degree. As you surrender flexibility through disuse, bone spurs called "osteophytes" form a hard edge to the joint, permanently limiting your range of motion. This severely limits the available joint surface area so that an enormous amount of force is concentrated onto a very small area. During your daily activities you may use only 25 percent of the cartilage that is available to you. You're apt to wear that joint out far more quickly.

Take the hip. As we get older and stiffer, our joints have an increasingly restricted range of motion. Imagine a billiard ball. Like the ball which fits into the hip socket, a joint is extremely smooth. The billiard ball gets worn evenly. Now imagine that you take the "eight" on the ball and just grind away at the number eight for days, months, and even years. That part will wear down more quickly. This can happen in your hip by focusing all of your activities such as walking, climbing, and running on one very small part of the joint's "ball." Increasing your range of motion allows you to concentrate that load over a far bigger area, often decreasing pain and increasing the life of a joint. Before starting this program, I was as stiff as they come, lucky to get my hands past my knees; now I can put my hands on the floor! Opening your joints is the key to self-healing.

Build Protective Strength

A relatively small increase in strength can lead to a large decrease in the risk of wear-and-tear arthritis. The most overlooked muscles in the body are those that protect our joints. These are called "periarticular" muscles and are the muscles that actually surround the joint. By strengthening them you stabilize the joint so that it doesn't self-destruct. You also improve reaction time and neurological connections so the joint can call upon the muscles it needs fast enough to protect itself. I'll show you a few simple exercises you can do in your home to build the strength you need where you need it the most to cut the pain and improve joint function. Restoring strength also helps to rehabilitate the cartilage, which requires regular compression for adequate nutrition and to stimulate repair. The little-known secret is that it is strength gained at the end of your natural range of motion that does the very most to build these protective muscles. If I'm pressed for time, I do one simple exercise that dramatically strengthens the muscles around my knees and hips. You can find this exercise, the Awkward Chair pose, on page 151.

Put Back the Spring

While doctors make a great deal out of aging joints, it's aging tendons, ligaments, and muscles that make us feel really old. What separates a twenty-year-old athlete from a fifty-year-old one is often the "springiness" of their muscles. The younger athlete's muscle is much more elastic. That means he or she can better absorb daily wear and tear, recover faster, and put in a superior performance. Muscle tightness in the groin and hip alone can accelerate deterioration of the knee. There's a whole chapter on putting the spring back in your step by increasing elasticity. Through a simple at-home exercise called a modified lunge, you'll build remarkable strength and stability with a complete range of motion.

Lighten the Load

Wear and tear is the only disease in which weight loss produces an immediate, noticeable clinical improvement. With each drop of ten pounds in weight, there is a greater than 50 percent reduction in pain! We profiled a 320-pound man with a severe disabling limp for a *Dateline NBC* broadcast. After he lost more than a hundred pounds, his limp, pain, and arthritis vanished. I see many people in their forties who put on an extra fifteen pounds and develop a limp. Weight loss delivers complete loss of pain. We'll look at the right foods for your joints, the ones that will spur the weight loss you need.

Play Joint-Friendly Sports

Aerobic exercise is terrific for your heart, your lungs, your brain, your waistline, *and* your joints. This chapter will help you find the sports that are best for you and your joints. It will also help you make those sports that are tough on your joints more joint-friendly.

Joint Nutrition

Joint cartilage is an ever-changing, dynamic living tissue that relies on the right package of nutrients to thrive. The appendix cuts to the chase and delivers the best and most reliable information on the supplements that can aid your aching joints.

The measures given in Part Two are the very best I've found anywhere after a long and arduous search. Good luck! You'll find that if you follow the remedies suggested in this book, you'll feel dramatically better, perhaps the best you have in decades.

PART ONE

Problems: What Causes Wear and Tear

1

Heel Pounders

Boom, boom, boom! Every night the sound of one jarring heel strike after the other bangs through the ceiling of our New York apartment. The noise makes it seem as if our upstairs neighbor is going to walk out on her husband for the last time. Ouch! The sudden, jarring sound is enough to wake the dead. So how do you politely tell your neighbor there's a problem? Try this.

Knock, knock, knock.
BOB: Hi! I'm Bob. I live downstairs. I'm very concerned about your wife.
HUSBAND: Oh, really. What seems to be the problem?
BOB: You see, we can hear her pounding across the floor in your apartment. Of course we're not concerned about the noise, we barely notice it. But I am concerned about the damage she may be doing to herself.
HUSBAND: Huh? What damage?
BOB: Well, you see, she's a pounder.
HUSBAND: A pounder? What's that?
BOB: There are two different kinds of walkers, pounders and sliders. Your wife, just from the sound we hear, is a four-star pounder. When she walks, she digs her heels into the

ground. Heel pounders are placing sharp, high loads on their knees. Over time that creates pain and over more time, may result in arthritis. I just thought you'd like to know. No use having your wife laid up.

HUSBAND: Gee, thanks.

BOB: No problem.

The conventional wisdom: A vigorous, heel-pounding stride is great exercise—and a good way to show you're in charge! The floor can easily be refinished.

The real deal: Don't worry about the floor; it's your joints you're killing.

REPETITIVE IMPULSE LOADING

The American Podiatric Medical Association says the average person takes eight to ten thousand steps a day. Fast, hard loading of the joints without adequate shock absorption is at the heart of joint wear and tear. That's the theory of Dr. Eric Radin at Tufts University School of Medicine who believes that repetitive impulse loading, or RIL, is required to damage cartilage and bone. Dr. Radin states, "It's not the amount of force, but the speed with which the load hits." Consider this analogy. Imagine driving fast over a bumpy dirt road with no suspension on your car. Every bump jars the frame and may damage your car or you! Slow the car down to a crawl, however, and even with the same heavy weight of the car's chassis on the frame, there's little damage because the speed of impact is reduced so drastically. It's the same with joints: slowly applied loads have little effect on the joint. Repeated rapid impulse loading, at the instant when your heel strikes the ground, produces joint damage. Why? Simply put, the very rapid application of load to the joint doesn't allow enough time for the muscles surrounding the joint or the joint tissues themselves to absorb the load. Be aware that the hard-and-fast landing is subtle and does not seem to enter the consciousness of most people.

On a scientific measuring device called a "force plate," this creates a very sharp spike. The rapidly applied force drives right through to your knees. Just think of it: with thousands of cycles a day and tens of millions cycles per year, you're damaging the joints and stiffening your tendons and muscles. You may well say, hey, no problem! That's what I've got cartilage for, to absorb the shock. Well, if that's the way you think, *big problem*! Contrary to popular opinion, cartilage and joint fluid have little shock-absorbing capacity. They're not good at attenuating peak loads.

As we'll see, well-controlled movement and strong, elastic muscles provide the best shock absorption.

Dr. Radin points out that you don't have to come down hard and fast, all you have to do is come down fast to create microdamage to the joints. The earliest detectable microdamage occurs in the bone underneath the joint cartilage in the form of microfractures.

Cheryl Riegger-Krugh, Sc.D., a physical therapist and associate professor at the University of Colorado Health Sciences Center, explains that bone is the fastest-adapting structure around a joint. The bone right under the joint cartilage adapts to this hard-and-fast loading by increasing in density. As a nice example, it's like playing basketball on a cement surface that does not give instead of on a wood surface that does. Playing basketball on a cement surface leads to more fatigue and soreness. Bone is able to adapt to the hard landings during gait from repetitive impulse loading. It can actually deform when it is loaded, and in deforming it provides a small amount of shock absorption. However, hardened, dense bone doesn't absorb the shock of landing during walking and thus the joint cartilage wears out as a result of pounding on the stiff bone underneath the cartilage. "The bone becomes much more rigid, and when it's more rigid, it doesn't give and the cartilage just keeps taking more and more of a beating because its underpinning isn't as resilient as it was," says Richard Ulin, M.D., clinical professor of orthopedics at Mount Sinai Hospital in New York City. Although the cartilage has no pain fibers, the bone has plenty, and the stiffened bone can cause real pain and disability.

If cartilage has little shock-absorbing capacity, what's the best way of absorbing shock? Well-coordinated, well-controlled muscle movement provides maximum active shock absorption. You'll find that as you learn well-coordinated, well-timed control of your limbs, you can significantly decrease, if not eliminate, pain and joint damage. Your muscles are your best shock absorbers. Learning to use them properly makes a world of difference.

The most recent research suggests that inappropriate loading may actually result in the production of molecules that signal the destruction of cartilage.

Dr. Riegger-Krugh asserts, "My own feeling is that the cause [of arthritis] is mechanical but the internal response in the body is biochemical."

MICROKLUTZINESS

Let's continue with my neighbor. Not wanting to risk getting a punch in the nose, I made my exit without telling her husband what I really thought of his wife. She was a klutz. I mean, she had "microklutziness." What's microklutziness? The correct timing and placement of the foot on the ground minimize the impact of a fast heel strike. That requires extremely exact muscular control. If you lack just a slight bit of precision, if you're just a little sloppy, your joint is hit with a sudden, jarring force for which it is not prepared. We use the term "micro" because to the eye you don't look like a klutz at all! You've probably experienced acute pain if you misjudged the height of a step, stair, or curb you've stepped off of. The microklutz experiences those jarring forces with every step, though to a lesser degree.

How do you get microklutziness? Dr. Radin states that most microklutziness is inborn. In some people, the fine neurological control necessary for precise movement goes hand in hand with muscular strength. If you have suffered a slight loss of strength as a result of an injury, disuse, or age, you might develop microklutziness. You may also suffer a *relative* loss of strength if you have gained weight and not increased your strength. This loss of strength is particularly bad when the muscle is the quadriceps, the muscle at the front of the thigh, since that is a key muscle in controlling the knee. Dr. Radin points out, however, that almost all the muscles play a role in coordinated movement. He believes that the loss of muscle coordination causes an individual to become a pounder.

This idea has been borne out in studies of patients with knee pain. When you're in optimal walking form, your muscles efficiently control the rate of descent of the foot as it approaches the ground. In people with knee pain or poor coordination, the ground is used as a brake. Ouch! Studies have shown that people who suffer from knee pain don't flex their knees at precisely the right time to protect their joints as their feet strike the ground. Simply put, they load their joints more rapidly and absorb shock less effectively. During heel strike they pound into the ground instead of sliding along it. This lack of appropriate deceleration of the leg is linked to minor neuromuscular incoordination, or microklutziness.

This kind of movement doesn't cause just knee pain. The force may be transmitted to the hip, says Dr. Radin. He points out that the hip is a joint that frequently doesn't "fit" quite right. The hip "doesn't have washers and spacers in it like the knee joint. The knee can take a little error and still be all right. The hip is a high-risk joint, and slight anatomic changes can really kick up trouble as you get older."

THIS IS NOT YOUR GRANDFATHER'S DISEASE

Okay, you may say, so I get arthritis when I'm eighty. So what? The sad fact is that microklutziness involves development of knee pain even in young adults. An ingenious study looked at the rate of loading on heel strike in a group of people who had the same walking cadence and speed. They found that those who already had knee pain hit the floor with a greater impact. The study concluded that "subjects with mild knee pain, possibly consistent with preosteoarthrosis, had a 37% higher loading rate of the vertical ground reaction force associated with heel strike." Quite simply, subjects with knee pain struck the ground faster and had a more violent follow through. Not only that, they absorbed shock less effectively, as evidenced by their landing with their knees straight and maintaining a straight knee after loading the forward foot while walking.

The most shocking aspect of the study was the subjects' age. They were in their *twenties*! Now is the time for them to make the change to prevent wear and tear, not when they're fifty or sixty years old and need a new knee joint! As we'll see, twenty-year-old basketball players already suffer thinning of the cartilage and changes in the underlying bone from the pounding they get while playing basketball.

While researching this book, I met hundreds of people, mostly women, who in their twenties and thirties already had knee pain from fast-and-hard heel strikes. Every one of them wore thin-soled, hard-heeled shoes and was a certifiable heel pounder!

SELF-TEST

Here's how to find out if you are a pounder. A highly sophisticated gait laboratory can tell for sure, but you can gather some clues on your own. There are more than a hundred gait labs in the United States. Temple University School of Podiatric Medicine's Gait Study Center in Philadelphia, the Hospital for Special Surgery Motion Analysis Lab in New York City, and Massachusetts General Biomotion Laboratory are among the best labs in the country and can be the most helpful in locating a good gait lab near you.

◆ **Do you walk loudly?** Walk across a wooden floor barefoot. Do you or your family or friends hear your heels pound? Do your neighbors complain? Compare your foot strike to others'. Is yours the loudest?

◆ **Does your calf muscle jiggle on heel strike?** Wear a pair of shorts during this test. Walk past a full-length mirror, such as one you might find in a health club. Walk with a forceful stride. Look to see if your calf muscle, also scientifically known as the gastrocnemius muscle, jiggles as you land. If you're a heel pounder, your calf will jiggle.

◆ **Look at your shoes.** Where are they worn? Do the heels wear down first? I found that mine do—right down to the sole! Do you have to replace your heels often? If your heels wear down very quickly, you may be a heel pounder.

◆ **Do you walk straight-legged?** Look at your stride in the mirror, say, on the wall in a gym or ballet studio. Is your knee straight when your heel hits the floor? Do you fail to bend your knee enough to absorb the shock? Do you put most of the shock impact on your bones rather than your muscles? Hold your thigh as you walk; feel how much your muscles contract normally, then try to flex your knee more. Feel the difference?

AT THE DOCTOR'S

Doctors familiar with this problem will be able to diagnose troublesome flaws in your gait quickly and effectively. Your best bet is a hospital with a formal gait lab or at least with a force plate.

Physical therapists or podiatrists with training in identifying the clinical signs of repetitive impulse loading are a more cost-effective and feasible way of identifying this problem.

Be aware that your joints may not hurt. That's because when joint degeneration begins, you don't feel pain since joint cartilage doesn't have a nerve supply.

SOLUTIONS

With osteoarthritis becoming an ever-greater problem among baby boomers, there needs to be more awareness of how to prevent it. Dr. Riegger-Krugh says, "It would be great if we could educate people to be aware of their movement and to let them know they can prevent this disease." Here are some simple steps you can take on your own.

1. Wear proper footwear. This is by far the easiest way to dampen the effect of heel pounding. Mario Lafortune, Ph.D., director of the Nike Sports Research Laboratory, says that virtually any kind of heel cushion will decrease the loading rate present at heel strike. See Chapter 8, "Fix the Flaws," for more on shoes. The right shoes can also help modify your gait.

2. Change your gait. Changing your gait can be a long and arduous process. Gait labs specialize in this; however, there are several simple suggestions to try before you invest in professional gait training.

◆ **Keep your hips level.** Use every opportunity to watch your hips when you pass a window or mirror. Do you see your hips bobbing up and down, or do they stay straight and level? You want to stay fairly straight and level so that there is less force on your heels as you land.

◆ **Use your knees.** Pounders have less maximum knee flexion and use their quadriceps for a shorter period of time after heel strike. Try to bend your knees more and use your quadriceps for a longer time to cushion your body weight as you land. If your knees are pretty much straight as you land, you're getting too little shock absorption out of your knees.

◆ **Use your feet.** Make a conscious effort to land on the outside of your foot and roll to the inside. This provides a substantial degree of shock absorption. The combination of proper knee and foot movement provides most of your shock absorption. In Chapter 3, "Fatal Flaws," we'll look at the different kinds of feet and how they are related to arthritis.

◆ **Float when you walk.** Make a conscious effort to walk as if you are on clouds and see if it decreases your pain! I have found that a combination of cushioned shoe inserts and shock-absorbing walking shoes go a long way toward helping you walk like this. Dr. Riegger-Krugh adds, "People need different kinds of cues, and I might use things like 'Think about walking on clouds' or 'Move as if you are walking across sponges or cushioned padding.' A patient recently used her own term: 'Think about walking on marshmallows.' The idea here is to walk with gentle heel landings. Try walking with a slight knee bend after your heel contacts the floor."

◆ **Land easily.** Dr. Riegger-Krugh says that just the suggestion that you land on your heels more easily can be enough to effectively change your gait and cut some of the forces.

◆ **Walk more slowly.** Dr. Radin believes that walking more slowly is a major way to cut out repetitive impulse loading. He points to the Chinese as evidence: "Old Chinese women walk slower than old Caucasian women. Osteoarthrosis is rare in Chinese women and common in Caucasian women." He counsels, "If you want to avoid arthritis, slow down if you have knee pain."

The evidence suggests that that's exactly what many people with arthritis do. Dr. Riegger-Krugh has tested people with advanced and painful knee osteoarthrosis. She has found that they load the leg cautiously following heel strike because loading is painful.

Dr. Radin also prescribes proper shoes: "What we do now to treat painful osteoarthrosis is, we prescribe jogging shoes that are nice and shock-absorbing and we tell them to walk slower. It seems to work." You do have to be careful, however, that when you slow your gait, you don't create a more harmful gait. You may, for example, be limiting the motion of a painful knee by placing potentially harmful loads on your hip joint. You do want to walk "normally" or, in other words, biomechanically correctly. The bottom line: If walking slowly results in an abnormal gait, speed up your gait until your stride feels correct.

3. Build stronger shock absorbers. Improve your onboard shock absorption. Muscle weakness leads to a bad gait, says Dr. Riegger-Krugh. Weakness, particularly in the quadriceps, is correlated with high repetitive impulse loading. So simply increasing the strength of your quadriceps can change your gait. Why? You'll have a real system of shock absorption to rely on—your muscles, not your bones and cartilage. Strong muscles can absorb more shock. Elastic muscles have more give and thus provide more shock absorption. Greater elasticity means that a muscle has more length over which to absorb shock. You can allow your knee to bend further and more quickly as you land to absorb the shock. The incidence of knee pain is lower in people using their quadriceps' strength to control the rate of joint loading as their heel strikes.

4. Improve your range of motion. I found that my own gait was tightly constricted by very tight knee and hip joints. If you improve your range of motion, your limbs will move more freely. You'll also be able to use your greater range of motion to absorb the load of foot strike. Chapter 9, "Restore Your Joints," includes a variety of simple yet highly effective exercises. By opening up your joints and breaking up the stiffness in the muscles and tissues around them, you can change your mechanics of walking substantially—from one that injures your joints to one that spares them. Knee and hip range of motion is obviously key, but so is the ankle joint, says Dr. Riegger-Krugh.

5. Decrease the load. Heel pounders slam into the ground with an initial force that is many times their body weight. More weight equals greater load. If that extra weight is in the form of body fat, it will also change your gait to a more awkward one. If your muscles are weak and you're overweight as well, you're doing even more damage to your joints. Many of us have become just too weak for the task at hand—at least to perform it biomechanically correctly—and when we carry extra weight we subject our joints to added strain. That's also true of carrying excess weight, from groceries to luggage. Buy luggage with wheels to decrease the load you have to carry for long distances. Chapter 12, "Lighten the Load," has more on how to shave off extra pounds.

A fierce battle is raging on every front. Not every researcher is hot on the idea of repetitive impulse loading as the root cause of arthritis. In fact, David Felson, M.D., M.P.H., at Boston University School of Medicine, one of the most prominent arthritis researchers in the world, is very cautious about saying that a deficient gait or heel strike might cause arthritis. However, he is pretty sure that once you have it, RIL will damage the cartilage over time.

What else might do the damage? As we'll see, wear and tear rarely results from a single factor. Pile one insult on top of another, and you have the formula for accelerating wear and tear and outright joint destruction. For instance, someone with a skeletal misalignment, such as bowlegs, can have excessively high joint contact pressure. Add RIL to that, and the odds of wear and tear are increased. Experts liken it to an organ failure. For example, heart failure may be the result of high blood pressure, heart attack, elevated cholesterol levels, smoking, and a bad diet. Like heart disease, joint wear and tear doesn't have a single cause. In the following chapters you'll find descriptions of other key problems that, when added to heel pounding, can accelerate the damage to your joints.

Dr. Riegger-Krugh concludes, "It used to be that arthritis was the nail in the coffin. The big message is, if you develop arthritis, there are a number of things that can change your functional status or your quality of life so that you may not need surgery or you may need it later and have a better quality of life in the meantime."

2

Stiff Man Syndrome

The big birthday with a frightening "0" at the end of it had arrived. I was stiff as a pretzel and just about as rickety. I'd always done lots of aerobic sports, weight training, and even a token amount of stretching. What had happened?

There's an ill of modern living that's almost never talked about—"stiff man syndrome"—and I'd come down with a wicked case of it.

What we suffer from, says Stephen J. Sontag, M.D., of Hines Veterans Administration Hospital and professor of medicine at Loyola University School of Medicine, is "muscle and tendon shortening which came about as a direct result of modern civilization." We consider it much more "civilized" to sit high on toilets and chairs. But look at parts of the world where even old men and women squat close to the ground to socialize, defecate, cook, and eat; people there suffer from arthritis much less. Try doing it! Most of us have completely lost the ability to squat; our leg muscles have become too stiff from lack of use. "Our modern lifestyle does contribute to shortening of our muscles. Sitting in our cars, at our desks with increasing computer use, in all likelihood leads to muscle shortening and unbalanced muscle pulls," says Gary Brazina, M.D., a Los Angeles–based sports medicine doctor and a fellow of the American Academy of Orthopaedic Surgeons.

Dr. Brazina says that staying in a static position for long periods of time without stretching or moving causes muscle shortening and subsequent imbalance.

Another key point, he says, is muscle shortening as a result of the modern lifestyle. One example: many women wear high-heeled shoes at work for hours each day. He especially cites cocktail waitresses in Las Vegas. Women who constantly wear high heels end up with shortening of the Achilles tendon. This can become so severe that they are unable to put their heels flat on the floor, he says.

The conventional wisdom: Use it or lose it.
The real deal: Most of us have already lost it.

Day in and day out, if we don't stretch them, our tendons and muscles get shorter and shorter. The tendons actually re-form thicker and shorter. Just as a highway department pours new concrete to repair a road, the body lays down new collagen in tendons. When it pours new collagen into a shortened tendon, it reinforces that shortening by making the tendon thicker. David Z. Prince, M.D., director of cardiac rehabilitation at Montefiore Medical Center in the Bronx, explains, "When muscles are not used, tissue fibroblasts become active rapidly and start to lay down new collagen in response to the lack of movement. Any unused muscle will become shortened, tight, and immobile very quickly—possibly within days. Why? It's a way of stabilizing an inactive or underused joint."

That tremendously restricts the motion of our joints. Dr. Sontag states that the price we pay for stability is reduced mobility. This also explains why it is so hard to stretch muscles back to their normal length and why a sudden stretch can cause a tear. In turn, our joints become constricted in their ability to move through their natural range of motion. We may initially mistake the stiffness in our joints, tendons, and muscles for arthritis. Over time, the resulting awkward motion patterns may damage the joint itself. That is, over time the stiffness produces abnormal forces on the joints and eventually leads to arthritis.

Even active people may gradually build up scar tissue in their muscles according to Topper Hagerman, Ph.D., of the Steadman Hawkins Clinic.

When traveling through rural Africa, I was faced with stiff man syndrome. I tried to squat but could do so only for a brief, exquisitely painful moment. I'd compromise by bending over at the waist with my hands on my knees for support. Travel through Africa, China, and India, and you'll see little arthritis. During a recent three-week trip to Yemen, where people squat to defecate, sit, and even pray, I found that hip replacement surgery is virtually unheard of. Bikram Choudhury of the Yoga College of India in Los Angeles claims that when he lived in India, there was no such thing as osteoarthritis of the hip. You'll see people squatting or sitting cross-legged. How many of us can do that anymore? Countries in which people routinely sit cross-legged on the ground have far less osteoarthritis of the hip than we have. Michael C. Nevitt, Ph.D., M.P.H., of the University of California, San Francisco, compared American women to Chinese women. Only 10 percent of American women aged sixty-five to seventy-four were able to squat to the floor and rise again. Compare that to an amazing 85 percent of Chinese women.

Do Chinese women get arthritis? Hip arthritis characterized by severe joint space narrowing was found in significantly fewer Chinese than in Caucasians. There were no cases of symptomatic hip arthritis in a study undertaken by Dr. Nevitt, comparing more than 1,500 elderly Chinese in Beijing to large population samples of Caucasians in the United States. Even the X-ray evidence of damage was much lower. Three Chinese women out of a thousand had X-ray evidence of wear-and-tear arthritis, compared to thirty-one out of a thousand American women. Researchers are looking for genetic and environmental reasons to explain the difference. The most intriguing, however, is stiff man syndrome resulting from a lack of squatting among Americans. Ironically, in this same sample, high rates of knee arthritis were found. Why? When you have pain in one leg, you favor the other, which puts the entire burden on that knee. That knee, then, is continuously traumatized. This means that the mechanics of gait is one key factor in the development of knee arthritis.

Let's look at arthritic hips. First there is pain, which emanates from the capsule that surrounds the joint. That pain inhibits normal muscle contractions, and the muscle becomes shorter and weaker. All of this is a *maladaptive* response to pain. Gently and carefully pushing through the pain and maintaining the natural range of motion helps to avoid the consequences. What consequences? Gregory Lutz, M.D., chief of physiatry at the Hospital for Special Surgery in New York City, says, "The biomechanics of how you walk are altered entirely. This may then *accelerate* the damage in and around the joint."

That may also be true of the knee joint. "The knee becomes stiff and limited in movement," says Colonel Gail D. Deyle, M.P.T. and chief of physical therapy at Brooke Army Medical Center at Fort Sam Houston in San Antonio, Texas. "As a result, it frequently doesn't straighten all the way out, it doesn't bend all the way, and the kneecap doesn't glide and move normally. Typically you also see patterns of muscle tightness that develop around an arthritic knee because it is limited in motion and function. Because the knee doesn't straighten all the way out when you walk, the muscles have to work harder to stabilize the knee. And as the muscles work harder, they actually increase the stress through the joint."

To me it's stunning how much loss we're willing to tolerate! If we'd lost as much heart function on a percentage basis, we'd be in a hospital ICU; this much liver function, we'd be on the wagon; this much lung function, we'd be hooked up to a respirator. It's just amazing that we let ourselves go that far! What's happening?

REPETITIVE TRAUMA SYNDROME

As we saw in Chapter 1, repetitive impulse loading has been linked to degeneration of the knee. That same repetitive motion also chips away at our muscles, tendons, and ligaments, creating a form of microtrauma. Over time, our muscles, tendons, and ligaments respond by scarring and growing shorter. The result is that we become stiffer and stiffer. The bottom line is that we need to do basic maintenance each day to undo the trauma of normal, everyday living. Just like a high-performance jet fighter or a helicopter needs hours of maintenance for each hour of flight, we too need maintenance to keep us "flying." That's especially true if you're a weekend warrior or if you're overloading your joints because of excess body weight—or, as is remarkably common, your thigh muscles are weak and unable to protect your joints properly during normal daily activities. Dr. Stephen Sontag even suggests that the diagnosis of "arthritis" is often incorrect. What we're really suffering from is stiff man syndrome! It was certainly true in my case. Sure, the X ray looks awful and arthritis is present, but that doesn't mean that the pain is being caused by the arthritis.

According to Dr. Sontag, even though there is inflammation, most patients with arthritis aches and pains generate them from the tendons and muscles that are continuously in a state of contraction from lack of stretching. When a muscle is not stretched out, it is tense, not relaxed. Constant tenseness squeezes the arteries that run through the muscle, thus diminishing the blood supply and oxygen to the joints and the rest of the muscle. The result of poor oxygenation is the buildup in the muscle of lactic acid, which in turn stimulates neurons to cause pain, muscle cramps, and more stiffness. Squatting, which is common in underdeveloped countries, is a natural stretching mechanism that keeps the extremities in good shape. Furthermore, stretching may even prevent disability from occurring after an injury. For example, after a traumatic accident, limping results as a natural mechanism to decrease the pain of movement. The limping in turn causes more muscle contraction, which in turn causes more limping. Thus a small injury (which all of us experience at one time or another) may well begin a vicious cycle of pain, limping, muscle contraction, more pain, more limping, and eventually a cane or crutches. In countries that squat, this downhill cycle is automatically interrupted numerous times each day—during defecation, socialization, and eating—and the acute traumatic event does *not* lead to a chronic disability.

Dr. Riegger-Krugh comments, "I think [higher chairs] were invented because people found they were easier to sit on and rise from . . . less muscle strength and joint range is needed to use them than to use lower chairs."

Very often the pain doesn't really come from the cartilage but from the stiffness in the joint capsule, the muscles, the tendons, and the ligaments—all of which may be fixable! But if you don't fix it, the pain will eventually become a permanent part of your life. You will damage your joints, and you will develop arthritis. For many of us pain is an early warning that it's time to do something. Unfortunately, we often take the road most traveled and allow ourselves to succumb.

TESTS: DO YOU SUFFER FROM STIFF MAN SYNDROME?

Even if you're an athlete, you may be startled by the degree of stiff man syndrome you suffer from. Typically, your anterior hip muscles and hamstrings are repeatedly shortened during activity. You likely don't even realize it. Let's take a look at your range of motion in key joints. The joints that are typically most restricted are marked with a bullet and are responsible for the primary disability in hip and knee arthritis. They're the heart of the stiff man most in need of correction.

Normal Hip Range of Motion

These are the average ranges of motion that doctors look for during their joint examinations.

Hip flexion: 110 to 120 degrees*
Hip extension: 10 to 15 degrees*
Hip abduction: 30 to 50 degrees*
Hip adduction: 30 degrees
Hip lateral rotation: 40 to 60 degrees*
Hip medial rotation: 30 to 40 degrees

Normal Knee Range of Motion

These are the average ranges of motion that doctors look for during their joint examinations.

Knee flexion: 130 degrees*
Knee extension: 10 degrees above the horizontal plane

A physical therapist can formally measure your joint range of motion using a device called a "goniometer." I've included the following series of tests you can use to informally determine what your range of motion is in your knees and hips.

The Hip

Hip Flexion Testing According to a recent article in the *Georgia Tech Sports Medicine & Performance Newsletter,* the hip flexors are one of the three most common muscle groups to cause problems. It recommends an excellent way to test your hip flexors to determine muscle group tightness: "Lie on your back and draw both knees to your chest. Continue holding the right knee to the chest while extending the left leg until it lies flat on the floor. Repeat the procedure to the other side. If you can't lay the extended leg flat, your hip flexors are too tight and in need of stretching exercises." *

---

* Reprinted with permission from the *Georgia Tech Sports Medicine & Performance Newsletter* 10, no. 3 (2001): 3.

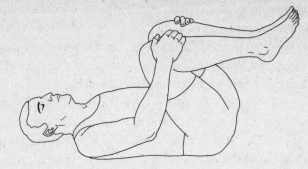

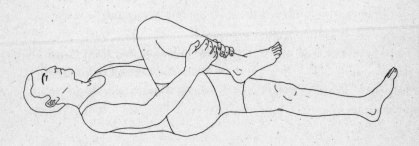

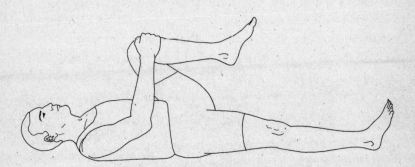

At a minimum, states Howard Nelson, a physical therapist in New York City, formally of the Hospital for Special Surgery and now with his own practice, you should be able to extend your hip about 10 degrees. When walking, our hips go through about 10 to 15 degrees of extension range of motion during the terminal stance. That is, just before the toe of the back leg comes off the ground while walking, the normal hip joint is in at least 10 degrees of extension. If you don't have that amount of motion, you may be moving too much from the next joint up, the lumbar spine.

Hamstring Flexibility Test In addition to hip flexors, another problematic muscle group, according to the *Georgia Tech Sports Medicine & Performance Newsletter,* is the hamstrings. It also recommends an excellent way to test * for hamstring group tightness. Lie flat on your back with the soles of your feet up against a wall and your knees bent at a 90-degree ankle. Now walk your feet up the wall until your legs are straight. Then pull your buttocks to the wall. You should be able to get your buttocks right up against the wall. If you can't get within eight inches, you have inflexible hamstrings.

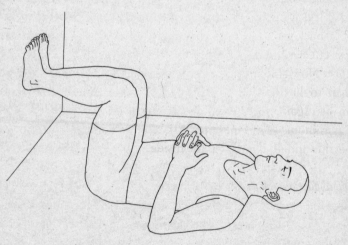

* Adapted with permission from the *Georgia Tech Sports Medicine & Performance Newsletter* (vol. 10, no. 3, December 2001).

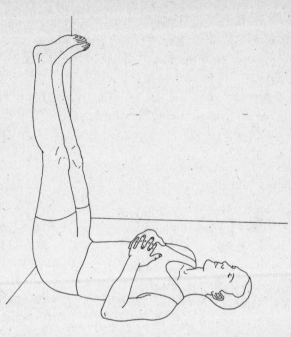

Hip Rotation Test Lie with your back flat on the floor and your legs straight. Nelson emphasizes that it is important to keep your back stable by utilizing your abs in order to make this stretch test effective. Also, be sure that your foot is kept in line with the knee. Now roll your feet to the outside. You should be able to roll them to the floor. That's external rotation. Now roll your feet to the inside. Again, you should be able to roll them close to the floor. At a minimum, your feet should be able to rotate 60 degrees to the outside and 40 degrees to the inside.

Hip Abduction, Adduction, and Extension

Hip Abduction Range of Motion Test Sit on the floor with your back stabilized against a wall and your feet together. Now gently move them apart as if you are attempting to do a split. Don't force your legs apart. You should be able to make at least a 90-degree right angle between your legs.

Hip Adduction Range of Motion Test Sit on the floor with your legs together. Now lift your left leg off the ground, high enough to clear your right foot. Keeping it straight, move it to your right, passing over your right leg. You should be able to move it 30 degrees. Repeat with your right leg.

Hip Extension Test Lie flat on your stomach on the floor. Keeping your left knee straight, lift your left leg off the floor. You should be able to extend your hip 15 degrees. Repeat with your right leg.

The Knee

Knee Flexion Test Lie flat on your stomach with both legs flat on the floor. Now try to bend your left knee and bring your left foot as close to your buttocks as possible. Repeat with your right knee. You can estimate your range of motion by determining how far past a 90-degree angle you can go.

Mark F. Reinking, physical therapist and assistant professor of physical therapy at Saint Louis University, says, "The normal range for the knee is 135 degrees. Knee flexion less than ninety degrees will interfere with most activities of daily living, such as transferring from sit to stand, going up and down stairs, and dressing. Given the motion requirements of daily living, knee flexion between 110 and 120 degrees is an acceptable range and is a suitable goal for rehabilitation after knee injury or surgery. However, participation in athletic activities requires normal knee range of motion."

Knee Rotation Test Your knee should also be able to rotate. Sit on a high chair or tabletop with your legs dangling over the edge. Kevin Wilk, physical therapist, emphasizes, "To be sure you aren't performing hip rotation, dorsiflex your foot [pull the toes up], which locks the tibia. Then hold down your thigh, and rotate your foot and shin in, then out. The lower leg should be able to rotate outward up to forty degrees and inward up to thirty degrees. This rotation is part of your shock absorption system."

Knee Extension Test Stand straight and lock your knees. Your knees should extend backward in the range of 0 to 10 degrees. Males will have a lower degree of extension. When your knees lock back to as much as 10 degrees past neutral, it is considered somewhat excessive and is called *genu recurvatum*. This is most common in females, who typically have looser joints and more flexible muscles than males do.

How did you do? If you are limited in your range of motion but have no existing arthritis or only mild arthritis and are less than sixty years old, strongly consider yoga as a way to restore your joints. If you are older or have more severe arthritis, you'll want a physical therapist to formally evaluate your range of motion and develop customized flexibility exercises for you. Why? You can hurt yourself by trying to force a badly damaged joint through an increased range of motion.

Dr. Stephen Sontag suggests several simple stretching exercises that mimic the effects of "squatting and frequently result in immediate and dramatic relief of symptoms." Before I began a course of yoga, I had a dull ache in my hip whenever I walked. My range of motion was severely limited in everything I did. For those of us with advanced stiff man syndrome, I believe that only a powerful solution—yoga, which really taxes the system—can truly reverse the condition. My first several yoga sessions were really painful and uncomfortable. Then I found the "immediate and dramatic" relief that Dr. Sontag spoke about. As you'll read in Chapter 9, I have regained all my youthful flexibility and range of motion, something I don't believe is possible with many standard stretching exercises. My own experience with the standard physical therapy handouts given out in doctors' offices was some pain relief but no real "fix." Yoga allows you to fix yourself. It allows you to regain the joint muscle and tendon flexibility that you have lost along the way but didn't deserve to lose, that range of motion that billions of people around the world never lose because they never stop squatting. After several months of yoga I found I could finally squat—and my hip pain was *gone*!

3

Fatal Flaws

My Apple G4 laptop was set off to one side of a narrow table at the Manhattan Sports Club dining room. I was trying to write a few pages of this book during a midweek lunch break. A pleasant woman approached me. "Gee, aren't you Dr. Bob? I just saw you on the *Today* show this morning." "Why, yes," I said. "What are you doing?" she asked affably.

"Working on a book on wear and tear."

As an afterthought I asked, "Say, do you have any joint pains?"

"Yes. In fact, my knee hurts." I asked her to put her feet together. She did. There it was! Her legs bowed out, leaving a space between her knees. She was definitely bowlegged.

"Is your pain on the inside of your knee?" I asked.

"Why, yes," she said with surprise.

"It's early wear and tear," I told her. "Your slightly bowlegged stance is part of the problem. Each time your heel strikes the ground, the impact forces strike the inside of your knee." Then I looked at her shoes, which had flat, hard leather heels. "Your shoes make that impact harder and faster." Almost with glee I thought, Here's an easy fix! A few changes now, while she was still in her twenties, would save her a lifetime of pain.

The conventional wisdom: It's age that destroys your joints.
The real deal: Fatal flaws will kill them!

The truth is that many of us have what I term "fatal flaws" in our skeletal structure. By "fatal" I don't mean they're potentially lethal, but they are serious skeletal malalignments that can lead to joint self-destruction.

Whether we're bowlegged or knock-kneed, these small variances from "normal" anatomy can increase the damage we do to our joints by direct wear and tear or by creating faulty movement patterns.

The big message is "Look for risk factors like skeletal malalignment and do something about it before you develop arthritis," says Dr. Cheryl Riegger-Krugh. "People may go to their doctors for some totally different reason, and the astute doctor would look at the alignment in your limb and ask if you have any pain and, if not, explain that that's because the cartilage hasn't been worn away yet and suggest that we do something about it before it happens. That would be just terrific."

Now, before you think of yourself as "abnormal," you should know that such flaws are quite common and even offer distinct advantages in certain sports. For instance, great ski racers are often knock-kneed, which gets them onto their inside turning edges more quickly. Great equestrians may be bowlegged, which allows them to sit a horse more securely. It's important to determine if you have any of the following fatal flaws that could accelerate damage to your joints, especially if you are a heel pounder or are overweight. The high impact described in Chapter 1 is bad enough, but "fatal flaws" can accelerate the damage. With day-in, day-out use, eventually something's going to wear out and break. Human beings put extraordinary stress on their frames. For instance, we walk an average of ten thousand strides per day over a nearly eighty-year life span.

Fatal flaws induce abnormal biomechanical loading, placing stresses and strains on the joints that are contrary to the way they were designed. These abnormal forces on the joints cause degeneration of the cartilage. This is not pure mechanical wear and tear.

There is an ideal alignment, says Howard Nelson. The further you are outside of ideal alignment, the more asymmetrical the forces are and the greater your risk of arthritis.

Nelson explains that the best analogy is a car. "When you are driving a car and your wheels are out of alignment, you can drive for fifteen thousand miles and then one day you will hear a repetitive clunking noise. What has happened is that fifteen thousand miles with a small asymmetrical load on your vehicle has made your tires wear unevenly and then you hear a clatter. The body is the same way. When a joint is ideally aligned, it moves in the center of instantaneous rotation. Each joint has a configuration where it moves in an ideal way. If that's not the case and you have it shifted to one side, you'll have asymmetrical wear on one or more of the surfaces and that causes increased pressure, wear of the cartilage, and pain."

KNOCK KNEES

"It really hurts. The doctor says there's a big divot." My mother rarely ever complained, even when a chip off her hip joint broke off. So I knew when she said her knee was sore she was in pain. She pointed with one finger to the outside of her knee. I then asked her to put her feet together. She couldn't. I said, "You're knock-kneed." She said, "I am *not* knock-kneed." I then replied, "Well, why can't you put your feet together?"

When she returned from her orthopedic surgeon, a superb joint specialist, she said he had told her that the cartilage was gone and there wasn't much to be done about it. I thought, Gee, there's *lots* you can do. We could brace your leg to put more pressure on the *inner* knee cartilage. Then I tested her leg strength. She could press only a few pounds. I looked at her flexibility. She could barely flex her knee past 90 degrees. Hmmm, I thought, I can fix *this*! Sure enough, in a couple of minutes, she'd improved her flexibility by 15 degrees with a mild quadriceps stretch. I promised her we could get to 80 degrees. By strengthening her knee, improving its flexibility and using a brace, I assured her, most of the pain would go away.

My oldest son is knock-kneed, too. It makes him a fabulous natural skier and a great tennis player. I advise him to stay away from hard heels and to wear shock-absorbing shoes. Knock knees were associated with a nearly fivefold increase in the odds of the progression of arthritis on the outside of the knee, as reported in the *Journal of the American Medical Association*. Knock knees leads to excessive rolling of the foot to the inside.

Self-Test

Stand in front of a mirror and bring your knees close together (touching). If your feet are still far apart, you probably suffer from *genu valgum* (knock knees). In lay language, the shape of your lower limbs will look like an hourglass.

Solutions

◆ **Use braces.** Braces have been developed specifically for bowlegs. Some physicians will try to modify an unloader brace (see page 31) for knock-kneed patients.

◆ **Wear shock-absorbing shoes.** (See Chapter 8.)

BOWLEGS

One of my best friends is a great horseman and snowboarder—but a terrible skier. Why? He is so bowlegged that he can't bring any significant force onto the inside edges of his skis. And watch him run, I swear it hurts just to watch! It looks as if his femur is about to break away from his lower leg and break to the outside on each step. His femur should be going fore and aft; instead it's clearly going from inside to outside. *Ouch!* Over time, that puts huge stresses on the inside of the knee. It's why I recommended that he not run.

The medial meniscus, the main passive shock absorber for the medial side of the knee, is at higher risk of injury and arthritis in bowlegged people. In general, arthritis affecting the medial compartment of the knee is ten times as common as the lateral compartment. Clinical professor of orthopedics Dr. Richard Ulin states, "It's probable that—and this is not based on science—significant angular deformity at the knee, such as excessive bowlegs or knock knees, will go on to an arthritic knee." Dr. Ulin found, in bowlegged patients, that "as they develop their symptoms, they notice that their knee becomes more and more bowed. And it does that as the wear and tear on the cartilage on the inner side accelerates. They lose cartilage, and then they are bone to bone. But as that happens their bowleg deformity increases. That leads to a terribly painful condition when the cartilage 'wears out.' " In fact, Leena Sharma, M.D., assistant professor at Northwestern University, found that the severity of knee arthritis was more strongly related to obesity in patients who were bowlegged. In fact, the more bowlegged the patients were, the worse their knees fared.

Interestingly, obesity appeared to play a smaller role in the disease severity of knock-kneed patients. The reason, Dr. Sharma explains, is that in the bowlegged condition, the load placed on the knee is concentrated more heavily on the inner part of the knee, which is more vulnerable to arthritis for a variety of reasons. With knock knees, on the other hand, the load is distributed more evenly across the inner and outer parts of the knee. Her study suggests that "people who are overweight and bowlegged may have more rapid progression of their knee arthritis."

If you're bowlegged, you have a fourfold increased risk for the progression of arthritis on the inside portion of the knee. As you walk, you naturally load up your lateral compartment first, then your medial compartment. The medial compartment is designed to be bigger since it usually takes more of the load. This compartment is gradually destroyed as the lateral movement of your leg becomes more and more pronounced. As we'll see, this force can be countered. Bowlegs can affect the feet as well and can contribute directly to the feet rolling to the outside or indirectly to the feet rolling to the inside.

Self-Test

Stand in front of the mirror with your feet close together, touching if possible. If there is still significant space between your knees, you are probably bowlegged. In lay language, the shape of your lower limbs will look like parentheses. Here's how you look for bowleggedness.

Draw a line from the center of the hip to the center of the ankle. The center of your knee should be on that line. If your knee is to the outside of that line, you are bowlegged.

The only definitive way to assess frontal plane knee alignment is with imaging techniques (e.g., leg X rays from the head of the femur to the foot).

Solutions

- ◆ **Play joint-friendly sports.** (See Chapter 13.)
- ◆ **Wear shock-absorbing shoes.** (See Chapter 8.)
- ◆ **Wear "unloader" braces.** These are a highly effective way of taking the pressure off the medial compartment of the knee, relieving pain and putting off the day you'll need to have the joint replaced by up to ten years. If your leg can be straightened out manually while you are lying on a table, you could be an excellent candidate for braces. A recent study of forty-two patients showed that the use of knee braces resulted in 35 percent less pain and 25 percent functional improvement. That's roughly the same pain relief you'd get with ibuprofen. Custom-made braces have been shown to be more effective than simple neoprene sleeves. These braces, such as the one made by Generation II Orthotics of Richmond, British Columbia, are called "unloader" braces. The technical name for it is a *Generation II unloader knee brace*. Its effect is immediate and significant, beginning as soon as the brace is put on. Moving X-ray pictures show that when the brace is in place, the joint actually opens. A custom-made osteoarthritis knee brace can run in the range of $1,300 to $1,500.

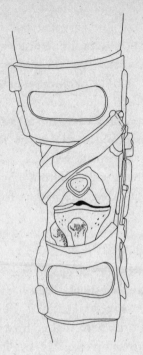

♦ **Wear neoprene sleeves.** Neoprene sleeves are the braces many of us have seen that fit snugly over the knee with a little window for the patella. A knee sleeve has no real mechanical effect on the knee and could not be expected to "unload" the knee. How does it work? It does so by giving patients a better sense of the position of their knees. That improved sense, technically termed "proprioception," may lead to their damaging their joints less by improving the overall coordination of their leg movements. Although not as effective as unloader braces, neoprene sleeves also decrease pain. Sleeves are also less cumbersome and easier to use. In addition, they warm the knee, which in itself may bring pain relief. A neoprene sleeve can run anywhere from $10 to $100, depending on its features and materials. The simplest ones are at the lower end of the price range; others have additional features such as patellar straps, sidebars, and hinges, which can increase the price significantly.

♦ **Use shoe wedges.** If you have already damaged the medial, or inside, part of your knee, you might consider using lateral wedges in your shoes. These wedges can decrease the load on the damaged part of your knee. The recent American College of Rheumatology recommendations for the medical management of osteoarthritis of the hip and knee state that "patients may benefit from wedged insoles to correct abnormal biomechanics due to varus deformity of the knee [knock knees]." Past research from the Center for Hip and Knee Surgery in Mooresville, Indiana, as well as various research done in Japan, reports that patients gain both pain relief and improved function with the use of laterally wedged insoles.

Fabian E. Pollo, Ph.D., director of orthopedic research in the Department of Orthopaedic Surgery at Baylor University Medical Center in Dallas, Texas, is well known for his biomechanically related studies that deal with conservative treatments, such as valgus (bowlegged) bracing and wedged insoles, for osteoarthritis of the knee. He suggests that wedged insoles be recommended to patients who:

♦ Are not overweight
♦ Have medial compartment osteoarthritis on just one side
♦ Have mild to moderate osteoarthritis
♦ Have no foot or ankle problems
♦ Have a knee varus angulation of less than 10 degrees (your M.D. can tell you this)
♦ Have no condition, such as diabetes, that results in loss of sensation in the lower extremity

Dr. Pollo states that there is no magic number for the degree of angulation for these insoles, but a good starting point is 5 degrees.

The clinical study done at the Center for Hip and Knee Surgery reported that when using lateral wedges, 38 percent of patients scored an excellent pain score, meaning they had little or no knee pain, while 50 percent had an improved pain score.

You can try this yourself either with a wedge you can buy at your local shoe store, shoe repair store, or pharmacy or with an orthotic made at a ski shop or high-end sports store. The standard orthotics available at the pharmacy can run from $4 to $20, while the custom-made ones can run from $50 to $150, depending on who makes them. If you notice considerable relief, you may want an experienced podiatrist or physical therapist to make a custom-made professional orthotic for you. The consensus among the podiatrists, physicians, and physical therapists interviewed for this book is to seek professional help for wedging, since you may actually cause additional problems by increasing the amount you pronate.

◆ **Wear proper shoes.** These will both reduce impact and control roll.

◆ **Lose weight.**

Both bowleggedness and knock-kneedness are risk factors not just for the development of arthritis, but also the progression of arthritis. If you have taken the tests for these conditions and determined that you have one of these fatal flaws, you have an important opportunity to prevent arthritis. If you already have arthritis, be sure to take these tests, since intervention now may still prevent the progression of the disease.

OLD INJURIES AND ILLNESSES

An old knee injury, even from high school, can increase the odds that you'll develop arthritis in that knee threefold, according to a study by Allan Gelber, M.D., M.P.H, Ph.D., and assistant professor of medicine in the Division of Rheumatology at Johns Hopkins University. Why? Because you may have developed small microfractures in your cartilage. High-impact activities may then wear away the cartilage over the years by hammering away at this flaw. You may also develop an unrecognized weakness in your quadriceps due to the injury, which may allow you to damage your joint inadvertently. Finally, abnormal biomechanics can create unusual and damaging forces that chip away at the site of an old injury. At highest risk are girls who have injured their knees in school sports. There are two ligaments that stabilize the fore-and-aft motion of the knee. The one most frequently injured is the anterior cruciate ligament, or ACL. A knee with a torn ACL often develops wear-and-tear arthritis. If the knee has been reconstructed, you can decrease that likelihood of advancing to arthritis but not eliminate it. The reason is that during weight bearing abnormal shear or sliding occurs, which slowly strips away the cartilage.

Players of football, soccer, lacrosse, basketball, and other team sports who have knee injuries are also at risk—specifically, those who have torn a ligament or who have small tears in the main cartilage, called the meniscus, which cushions and separates the bones of the upper and lower leg. (The highest injury rate, surprisingly, may come from volleyball.) The link between knee surgery in which the meniscus is removed and knee osteoarthritis is also well documented. According to Dr. Gelber's study, the cumulative incidence of knee osteoarthritis by age sixty-five was 13.9 percent in participants who had suffered a knee injury during adolescence and young adulthood and 6 percent in those who did not.

It's not just sports; your job may also put you at risk. If you do a lot of heavy lifting and climbing of stairs or ladders, you're at greater risk of developing arthritis. The other occupational group that suffers lots of arthritis of the knee? Physical education teachers! No kidding! Even though they smoked less, weighed less, and were more active, they ended up developing knee disorders. That made me a convert to the idea that the wrong kind of overactivity can be a bad thing!

Old illnesses as well as injuries can also put you at risk. Go over your medical history to determine if you have had any of the following illnesses or injuries, arranged by age:

Hip Disorders

Check your medical records to determine whether you suffered from any of these conditions as a child. Each of them increases the risk of arthritis. Early diagnosis is vital to prevent further damage to your joints.

◆ **Infants:** Developmental dysplasia.
◆ **Children four to ten years of age:** Legg-Calvé-Perthes disease. The greater the deformity of the femoral head, the worse the long-term outcome.
◆ **Older children:** Slipped capital femoral epiphysis.
◆ **Young to middle-aged adults:** Osteonecrosis.
◆ **Older adults:** Degenerative joint disease or hip fracture.

If when you walk you have either a toe-in or toe-out gait, you may have had a previous hip disorder.

Knee Disorders

◆ **Children three to eight years of age:** Blount's disease.
◆ **Teens, people in their early twenties, and women:** Patello-femoral (kneecap) disease.
◆ **Early teens to the mid-fifties:** Meniscal tears.
◆ **Teens to the forties:** Ligament injuries.

A good clue that you're in trouble is the development of pain and a "crunching" sensation or sound in the joint. After learning about the link between sports and arthritis, I've become much more careful with my own children, since the consequences are lifelong. You may be the hero of the day in a football game at age fourteen but pay the price at age thirty. Protect your kids! Encourage noncontact sports to reduce the risk of injury. If your kids play soccer, football, lacrosse, or other sports that have a higher risk of joint injury, insist they have the proper skill level and conditioning to compete safely. The conditioning exercises in this book will take them a long way toward doing that! My own idea is that if you are fabulously talented at a sport or love it more than life itself, do it! With great strength, skill, agility, and flexibility training you may well protect yourself. But if you're just going through the motions, find a "life" sport that doesn't have the same risks and that you can enjoy into old age.

Solutions

- ◆ **Play joint-friendly sports.** (See Chapter 13.)
- ◆ **Wear protective footwear and braces.** (See Chapter 8.)
- ◆ **Use joint-protective drugs.** (See Chapter 6.)
- ◆ **Avoid chronic use of pain relievers.** These can mask the problem.
- ◆ **Do yoga and stretching exercises.** If you do joint-unfriendly sports, be willing to take the time to recover with a full yoga and stretching routine.
- ◆ **Have an orthopedic evaluation done.** This will determine whether you need corrective surgery or even debridement of the knee to remove excess pieces of cartilage that may be floating in the joint.
- ◆ **Have an MRI done.** This can determine the extent of any damage from old injuries.

STIFF JOINTS

Stiff joints encumber the way you move and, in doing so, set up faulty biomechanics. That faulty gait can then accelerate the damage you do to your joints. The best example is the hip, where most of the reduced range of motion comes from joint stiffness, not from damage to the joint. The self-test in Chapter 2 will allow you to determine if your range of motion is restricted.

Solutions

- ◆ **Do yoga.** (See Chapter 9.)

37

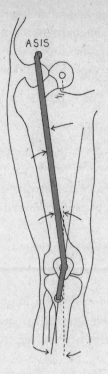

ASIS

LARGE Q ANGLE

The Q angle is the angle formed by the lines between the anterior superior iliac spine (ASIS, the sharp point in the front of your pelvis) and the middle of the kneecap and the line between the middle of the kneecap and the tibial tuberosity (the protrusion on the front side of the tibia just below the kneecap).

A large Q angle may be associated with anterior knee pain and chondromalacia of the patella in young women. A greater Q angle theoretically places greater lateral stress on the kneecap, causing poor tracking of the kneecap within the femoral groove. However, the biggest risk of a large Q angle is when it is linked to excessive pronation, believes Patrick J. Nunan, D.P.M., podiatrist and president of the American Academy of Podiatric Sports Medicine.

"That could cause any biomechanical deformities that start in the feet and actually put excessive strain on the hip." Read more about overpronation on page 45.

LOOSE JOINTS

Lax knee ligaments can be a factor in arthritis. Ligaments stabilize joints such as the knees. If these ligaments are not reasonably taut, there can be excess "play" in the joint. For instance, the knee may be prone to wobble to the inside or outside if the collateral ligaments, along the outside and inside of the knee, are lax. Some doctors believe the laxity in itself doesn't contribute to arthritis but could predispose a person to an injury, which, in turn, will predispose him or her to arthritis. However, hypermobile joints can lead to mechanically unsound limb positions, which, on a repeated basis, may lead to arthritis. Women may have a higher degree of lax ligaments than men.

Dr. Cheryl Riegger-Krugh adds, "I think the laxity and the shear can cause joint degeneration."

UNEQUAL LEG LENGTHS

Another fatal flaw is having different leg lengths. Over time, this can create damaging stresses. In fact, most of us have unequal leg lengths. What we're talking about here is leg-length discrepancies that create extra shear and stressing forces on the joint. Those forces can damage both knees and hips. Jeffrey A. Ross, D.P.M., podiatrist and assistant clinical professor at the Baylor College of Medicine, says, "It's amazing to see not just so much arthritis but people who probably had limb-length differences that were never diagnosed their whole lives who later on had destroyed knees and hips because of wear and tear due to the fact that their legs were asymmetrical." Do you have curvature of the spine, or scoliosis? This can create a pelvic tilt, which then creates a functional limb-length difference.

Self-Test

You'll need a friend's help with this one.

1. Stand against a wall in your bare feet. Have your friend see if one hip is higher than the other. Then locate the bony protuberance on the front of the hip, called the anterior superior iliac spine. Determine if one is higher than the other.

2. Have your friend watch you walk to see if one shoulder is lower than the other. Paradoxically, the shoulder that is higher may be on the same side as the shorter leg. That's because it may compensate for the pelvic tilt on the side of the short leg.

3. Lie flat on a table with your legs straight and together and your arms by your sides. Have your friend measure from the bony protuberance at the front of your hip (called the anterior superior iliac spine) to the prominent bone protruding from the inside of your ankle (called the medial malleolus) with a tape measure. Any difference between the two measurements means you may have a leg-length discrepancy. Since other hip or foot problems can create an apparent discrepancy, have a health care professional evaluate you if you detect a difference in length on this self-test. Physical therapists deal with this problem frequently.

Solutions

Add a ⅛-inch heel lift to your shoes. This may be one that is removable—that is, you put it into your shoe under an orthotic, or you can have the lab (or whoever is making the orthotic) incorporate a ⅛-inch lift in the rear foot post of the device itself as a permanent fixture. Even if it seems to work, be sure to check with your doctor since in certain patients it may cause the foot to roll excessively to the inside.

HIP SHAPE

The ball of your hip can vary in diameter from 42 to 56 millimeters. David E. Krebs, PT, Ph.D. in pathokinesiology and physical therapy at the Massachusetts General Hospital, says, "The pressure can increase *tenfold* within those joints whose ball has a small diameter. Where there is already thinning, it is worn away faster." In another pathological condition called "hip dysplasia," the peak contact is located more to the outside and in front, increasing wear and tear. The hip's configuration and shock-absorbing qualities may also be changed by disease and lead to localized arthritis. Ask your doctor to check your medical record for these conditions:

◆ Fracture of the femoral head
◆ High-dose corticosteroid therapy treatment
◆ Pancreatic disease
◆ Alcoholism
◆ Sickle-cell disease
◆ Caisson disease
◆ Diabetes
◆ Gaucher's disease
◆ Damage to the nerves innervating the hip muscles

I was particularly surprised to learn that bursitis or even a strained muscle can cause uneven wear of the hip joint. For instance, if your right hip hurts from bursitis, you'll tend to lean more toward the left, which can cause undue wear on the left side. Should your doctor order an X ray, here are two other deformities he or she will be looking for:

◆ **"Pistol grip" deformity.** In this condition the upper end of the femur bone looks like the handle of a derringer; hence the term "pistol grip." This can lead to early arthritis of the hip and the knee and require joint replacement at a young age.
◆ **Femoral neck angle.** The femoral neck angle is an important factor in hip stability and normal walking. An abnormal angle can lead to disabling arthritis of the hip and knee in adults.

ABNORMAL GAIT

"An alteration in your normal gait may be a significant predisposing factor to the development of hip arthritis," writes Kevin Sims of the Department of Physiotherapy, University of Queensland, Australia. "The abnormal gait may create abnormal forces on your hip joint, that becomes the primary driving force of the destructive process." This abnormal gait may result from problems anywhere from the lower spine to the foot.

EXCESS BODY WEIGHT

Obesity changes gait patterns and loads on joints such as the knees. The extra weight also has a direct damaging effect on the joint. For more on this, see Chapter 5.

FATIGUE

It may seem odd to think of normal muscle fatigue as a fatal flaw because it's only a temporary condition. But when a muscle begins to fatigue, it can cause an abnormal gait. Simply put, when the muscles are fatigued, the joint may not work properly. As muscle fatigue sets in, the muscle is overloaded and eventually the joint will overload itself to spare the muscle. If you already have joint damage, you put your joints at further risk if your muscles are fatigued. I always used to exercise even when my muscles were extremely fatigued. I still do, but not activities such as hiking, running, or other sports that place high loads on the joints to begin with. I'll stick with cycling.

THE WRONG SHOES

There may be absolutely nothing wrong with you but your shoes. The wrong shoes can "fake" an abnormality. For instance, take a shoe with a very soft midsole. When your foot rolls in as you walk, it puts pressure on the inside of the midsole and because the midsole is soft, it crushes it, simulating a structural abnormality. If you bought the shoes to fix a problem, you're now facing double trouble! You bought them to absorb shock but end up creating powerful and unusual forces in your foot.

Hard Leather Heels

They look great on light casual shoes but provide the least cushioning and the greatest shock to your knees. Wear them sparingly! Flat leather heels pack even more punch. If you love them, wear running shoes to get to work or an event, then switch!

FEET

Physical therapists such as Kenneth Holt, Ph.D., PT, at Boston University, spend their lives looking at dozens of different abnormalities of the foot. "I've seen people twenty-five years old with fairly serious osteoarthritis," says Dr. Holt. "You can nail the mechanics right down to a particular kind of foot problem." But of them all, there are two foot abnormalities that cause the most wear and tear to the body. The first causes excessive motion and/or poor timing of joint motions, the other too little. They are the "destructive foot" and the "claw foot." As a youth you may have noticed few problems, but with age, the foot begins to weaken and deteriorate and the arch to collapse. So a flat foot or even a mildly flexible flat foot early on in life can worsen as you get older. Before you plunge ahead with the rest of this chapter, do this simple test to see if you may have a problem.

Self-Test: What Kind of Foot Do You Have?

Set a piece of paper on the floor. Now wet your foot. Assume a normal stance, then place your wet foot on the piece of paper or any other surface on which you can leave a good imprint of your foot, such as a cement floor.

◆ Normal foot

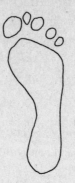

Normal foot

◆ If you see a big, broad-based footprint, you may be a high roller. Remember, your foot needs to be completely flat on the wet foot test to be a true high roller. Otherwise you may simply have a low arch.

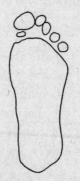

High roller (overpronation)

◆ If you see only a very narrow, outside edge of your foot, you may have a rigid, cavus foot.

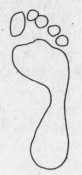

Cavus foot (rigid)

If you have either of these types of feet, read on!

Overpronation, A.K.A. the "Destructive Foot"

"The destructive foot," says Dr. Kenneth Holt, "produces forces that are huge and go through all the joints. Some people end up with these arthritic changes that go right through the whole system. It's the one I see most in my practice because it's the most devastating." The forefoot varus abnormality has been termed the "destructive foot" for the chronic and sometimes debilitating injuries it can cause throughout the body.

During a normal stride, there is a normal inward roll of the foot, allowing it to act like a shock absorber when the foot comes into contact with the ground. This inward-rolling motion is called "pronation." However, this rolling is supposed to occur for only a split second, until the end of the stride, when the heel begins to lift off the ground. If the rolling is prolonged, you're a high roller! Let's take an in-depth look.

What It Does

The destructive foot's natural position before it strikes the ground is rolled too far to the inside, the foot inverted with the sole facing the opposite foot. That means that the outside of your heel strikes the ground first, which is normal. As you place your foot on the ground during a normal stride, the destructive foot comes down and rolls in. Since you are hitting on the outside of the foot, the foot has to roll a great deal more before the stride ends. This generates more and more force, more and more velocity. Over time the structures that support your foot's shape and position start to break down; the joints, ligaments, and muscles that support your arch all lose that capacity.

You may first encounter more minor problems, such as shin-splints or scarring of tissue along the bottom of the foot, called plantar fasciitis.

The destructive foot can cause far more serious problems higher up in the body because as your stride ends, your foot is still trying to roll your lower leg in, while your lower leg is trying to roll out. Those two opposing forces produce a tremendous torsion in the knee joint. That torsion leads to a very tight joint capsule. Dr. Holt explains that it actually starts to break down the supporting structures of the knee joint. The damage is done to the joint surfaces between the upper leg and the kneecap and between the upper and lower leg. The resulting knee pain is often on the inner side of the knee, he explains. Sometimes the inward forces that are created in the lower leg even get carried through to increase twisting movements in the hip and back.

If the knee joint is very, very stable, the forces are carried through from the foot through the lower leg, through the thigh, and then into the hip. That produces excessively high forces in the hip. The destructive foot can also throw your posture off, creating excessive forward body lean, which may result in a swayback.

Another major consequence is called "iliotibial band syndrome." The iliotibial band is a ligament that runs between the upper and lower leg, rubbing against the lateral side of the femur with each step. The angled forefoot leads to a tightening of the lateral collateral ligament. This condition is characterized by inflammation and pain on the lateral side of the knee. A lack of flexibility and strength in this ligament or "band" contributes to the pain. The pain typically occurs after a mile of running and diminishes after stopping. With excessive heel strike, this lateral impact and tightening go all the way up the chain, from heel to hip.

If you have been diagnosed with one of the following, you should consider overpronation as a cause.

♦ **Plantar fasciitis.** A painful condition of the tendons and ligaments on the sole of your foot.

♦ **Shinsplints.** Pain along your leg bone or shin.

♦ **Medial knee pain.** Pain on the inside of your knee.

♦ **Neuromas.** A foot condition caused by an abnormal function of the foot that leads to bones squeezing a nerve, usually at the ball of the foot between the third and fourth toes. Neuromas are associated with pain, swelling, and/or inflammation of a nerve. Symptoms of this condition include sharp pain, a burning sensation, and even a lack of feeling in the affected area.

♦ **Bunions.** A protrusion of the big toe joint, also known as the metatarsophalangeal joint.

♦ **Hammertoes, sometimes called clawtoes.** A condition when the toes become crooked and bent and start to buckle under, causing the joints to protrude.

♦ **Lateral ankle sprain.** An ankle sprain of the structures on the outside of the ankle.

CLAW FOOT

The other major foot type that can cause problems is the high-arched, "rigid" or "cavus" foot. The normal roll of a foot during the landing phase of a normal gait, known as pronation, provides substantial shock absorption. The rigid foot does not roll enough to provide good shock absorption. If you have a rigid foot, you're getting too little shock absorption, and over time that can inflict real damage. "If you lose pronation, you've lost a lot of your shock-absorbing capacity," confirms Dr. Gregory Lutz of the Hospital for Special Surgery. And where does the shock usually go? Dr. Patrick Nunan states that it sometimes affects the feet, but usually the shock travels right up the chain into the knees, hips, and lower back. The foot also acts as an adapter to the varied surfaces we walk on.

A rigid foot has a lesser ability to adapt, say, as you walk over rough terrain, because it can't roll enough. One tip-off that you may have a cavus foot is lateral knee pain or even back pain.

"I've seen more and more people with the aging population coming in with arthritis in their back," states Dr. Nunan. People with high-arched feet take a real pounding. That's why they have lower leg pain, knee pain, hip pain, and low back pain. A digger with a heavy heel strike will have extra misery. What kind of misery? Metatarsal stress fractures, ankle sprains, lateral knee pain, even hip dysfunction, says Dr. Jeffrey Ross.

Since the big problem is poor shock absorption, a bad combination for a cavus foot is a heavy heel strike, which creates large, damaging forces.

People with high-arched feet don't tend to go into running because they find out at an early age that they develop pain. Only in writing this book did I discover my own high-arched foot. Now I understand how I developed early arthritis: thousands of miles of walking, hiking, and running with little shock absorption! Just knowing I have the problem has already made a big difference. The right shoes and a modified style of walking have helped tremendously.

OTHER SYMPTOMS

Here are some other pretty good clues that you may have a foot problem. A good podiatrist or orthopedic foot surgeon is your best guide for a final diagnosis.

◆ **Calluses.** Think of calluses as a problem of excess friction or pressure. *Where* your calluses occur may be a tip-off.

◆ **High rollers/overpronators:** Look for calluses on the big toe itself.
◆ **High-arched foot/claw foot:** You may see calluses across the entire ball of the foot.

◆ **Shoe wear.** Shoes may give you several very valuable clues. First, look for signs of wear:

◆ **Wear near the big toe.** This shows that your foot is rolling inside to the extreme before you push off and is a tip-off that you may be a high roller. Look at your shoe sole, and you'll find that it is most worn in the same place you'll find calluses on your foot.

◆ **Wear along the outside of the heel.** You may be slamming your foot down too quickly and rolling your foot too fast from outside to inside. Do you land on the outside of your foot only to roll all the way over to the inside and then press off on your big toe? You may be a high roller!

◆ **Wear along the outside of the entire sole.** This is typical of the high-arched cavus foot. While high rollers may have different patterns of wear, the cavus foot is pretty consistent in terms of wear.

◆ **Asymmetrical wear.** Look for harder wear on one shoe than the other. If one shoe wears harder than the other, it may indicate a leg-length discrepancy. It could also mean you are taking too long a stride with one leg if you find wear in the center of one heel and to the side of the other heel.

◆ **Shoe test.** Take the shoe, put it up high on a flat surface, and stand behind it at eye level. Look from the back of the shoe to see if it is perpendicular or not. If you see that the shoe is distorting either laterally or medially and the lateral wear is excessive (particularly to the outside of the shoe), you should be suspicious. If your shoe is worn in either direction, your first sign of trouble may be shinsplints!

Since shoes may wear differently, look at several pairs. Shoes can be tricky. So if you see excessive wear, it's a clue, but don't pin your whole diagnosis on your shoes!

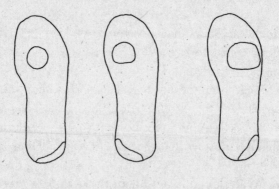

Normal foot   *High roller*   *Cavus foot*

Solutions

◆ **Use sports orthotics.** I love these because they're highly pliable, comfortable, and functional. I use a brand called Superfeet orthotics, produced by Northwest Podiatrics, (800) 634-6618, because they can be custom fit in a shop in about twenty minutes. I use them in my running, tennis, and even cycling shoes. They produce a stable footbed that prevents excessive roll of the foot to the inside or outside.

◆ **Wear the proper sports shoes.** There are specific shoes that counter the roll of the high roller and cushion the shock for the cavus foot. (See Chapter 8.)

◆ **Play joint-friendly sports.** Choose low-impact sports from Chapter 13.

◆ **If you are a high roller, consider using a wedge inside your shoe.** "In Japan they use orthotics for the treatment of OA of the knee and hip. The use of orthotics can change the ground reaction force with heel strike so that the forces that the knee, hip, and spine see can be diminished," says Dr. Gregory Lutz. Be aware, however, that improperly fitted wedges can sometimes cause additional problems because they may introduce a new flaw.

◆ **See a podiatrist or physical therapist.** If you have complicated foot problems that don't go away with good sports shoes and sports orthotics, you're probably due for a trip to a first-rate sports podiatrist or a physical therapist specializing in orthotics. Since flawed feet can reach so much higher up into the skeleton—to the hips, knees, and even back—it's worth making an effort to get to the root of the problem.

COMBINATION PROBLEMS

The human body has a remarkable ability to accommodate. Dr. David Krebs says that the human body is so plastic and so adaptive that a single insult is easily compensated for. A single biomechanical imperfection may not lead to pain, but combined forces could cause trouble. For instance, a female, knock-kneed digger who wears wide high-heeled shoes is much more likely to get into trouble than most!

Howard J. Hillstrom, Ph.D., director of the Gait Analysis Study Center at Temple University Podiatry School, adds, "Malalignments in the lower extremity rarely travel alone. You may have uncovered one problem only to miss another." He warns that inappropriate therapy can exacerbate the problem, increasing stresses to the overloaded region of the involved joint." Dr. Hillstrom's study center is one of the first to look at combinations of conservative treatments such as wedging and bracing. For example, its staff members look at using combinations of valgus bracing and medial wedging. Currently a few pilot studies are being completed, and the results look promising.

4

The Weak Link

What's *your* weakest link? Are you a hand stander? That's a person who has to place both hands squarely on the arms of a chair and then press down firmly to stand up. The hand stander may feel strong enough when standing up, but the strength comes from the arms, not the legs. The fact is that the hand stander hides leg weakness by relying on the arms. Walking down a flight of stairs, the hand stander again relies on the banister or even drops each hip toward the next step to make up for weakness in the worst possible place, the thigh muscles. This is not your grandfather's problem. Many of us, from the fittest weekend warriors to the most active supermoms, have undetected muscle weakness that predisposes us to further injury, significant wear and tear, and early arthritis. For many of us, it's the biggest risk of wear and tear, yet it's never occurred to us that we have a weak link.

The conventional wisdom: I'm strong!
The real deal: Unperceived weakness is at the heart of wear and tear.

Quadriceps weakness is one of the earliest symptoms reported by arthritis patients and often precedes the development of knee pain and disability. Amazingly, this leg weakness is a better determinant of pain and disability than even X-ray changes. Michael Hurley, Ph.D., an osteoarthritis and rehabilitation expert at King's College, London, confirms that "an X ray will actually tell you very little about the actual disability that the patients have. But if you measure somebody's muscle strength and they are weak, then they are very much likely to be disabled."

For that reason, quadriceps weakness is a key screening test for your risk of wear and tear.

None of this may seem very startling to you, but it has been a revolution in thinking for doctors. "Everyone has been in the mindset that it's the joint damage that causes the muscle weakness," adds Dr. Hurley. There had been little suspicion that the muscles weakened first, directly contributing to the onset and progression of arthritis. Here's how.

AGING

We all lose muscle with age, beginning around age forty. "Cross-sectional studies have shown reduction in muscle strength with age in both men and women," reports Kenneth Brandt, M.D., professor of medicine and head of the Rheumatology Division at Indiana University School of Medicine in Indianapolis. The decline in muscle strength with aging can be attributed to the loss of muscle and the muscle's capacity to generate force. That loss accelerates at age fifty, and by age eighty we've lost approximately 40 percent of our total skeletal muscle mass. This accounts, in part, for the decline in muscle strength seen with aging. Some of this decline can be avoided with weight training.

Now let's take a closer look at the quadriceps. Why are the quadriceps so important? Quite simply, the quadriceps act as a brake. As your leg descends during a normal stride, the quadriceps slows the heel as it approaches the ground. Once your heel hits the ground, your quadriceps are shock absorbers that dissipate potentially damaging forces before they hit the joint. With weakened quadriceps, the load goes straight to your joint as your heel lands on the pavement. Strong quadriceps also guard against sudden sharp forces. If you have softened or damaged cartilage, this protection is even more important. Weak muscles present a clear and present danger to the joints! At this point, if you're like me, you're saying, "Naw . . . not me, I'm fine!" But it's not easy to know if you are weak. Why? If you have strong buttock and calf muscles, they will compensate for your quadriceps weakness but not enough to protect your joints. Trust me, you'll go through life thinking you're strong as a bull but silently suffer from an undetected weakness that leaves your joints vulnerable. Quadriceps muscle weakness plays a primary role in knee pain, disability, and progression of joint damage in knee arthritis.

SHEAR FORCES

The quadriceps also function as stabilizers, which can dampen torque or shearing forces. Even more damaging than a sharp impact is a twisting force. That's what often damages cartilage when you suffer a sports injury. But you may be applying those shearing forces every day if you have lax joints or ligament injuries or if you are slightly uncoordinated in the way you walk, what we call a microklutz.

Shearing forces are produced when adjacent surfaces slide across one another. As with the knee, the shearing force is caused by the shifting of the tibia and the femur. This is caused by the strong contraction of the quadriceps as in the open-chain knee extension. This force occurs in the front of the knee and places a lot of stress on the ACL.

POWER

William Kraemer, Ph.D., at the University of Connecticut, draws a sharp distinction between strength and power: "Strength is force exerted at slow speed. Power is the ability to summon force quickly. Power is more important in daily life. If you slip on ice while carrying a bag of groceries, it is a surge of power that allows you to shift and keep your feet." Power provides the ultimate protection for your joints. As we'll see, the movement and balance you will gain from more functional exercises such as squats, combined with adequate power, are your ultimate goals. Dr. Kraemer says, "In a training program you need to train both components of the equation: strength to keep your force capability high and then rapid force development to improve power."

COORDINATION

Hand in hand with muscle weakness go a loss of position sense and the necessary reflexes to protect your knee joint. Curiously, Dr. Hurley points out that it may not be the loss of strength so much as the loss of reflexes that poses the greatest danger: "If something happens to the muscle first, as soon as those protective reflexes are compromised in any way, you haven't got the protection of the joint." Here's a practical example. You're walking over some rough ground and misjudge your step because you're not exactly sure where your knee is. That's a loss of position sense. Now you try to react to your clumsy misstep but your muscles can't respond quickly enough. Weak muscles are fatigued more readily and lead to excessive joint movement and instability, which elicits pain and gives rise to rapid, jarring loading of the joint. As your foot lands on the ground, you don't have the strength to protect your joint either. You feel a twinge of pain as you grind into your cartilage, chewing it up as you land.

FATIGUE

I'd just taken the ten-hour overnight flight from Harare, Zimbabwe, to London. I went right to the basement health club of

London's Grosvenor Hotel and began to pump away on the Stair-Master. It just didn't feel right. My joints were sore during the workout and afterward. Why? Dr. Joseph Feinberg, a physiatrist at the Hospital for Special Surgery in New York, says, "Although you may be strong, fatigue can lead to muscle overload. Fatigue can also lead to altered biomechanics and injury to other muscles or other structures such as the ligaments, joints and bones." Whether after a long flight with no sleep or a marathon, joints are especially vulnerable to damage when you are fatigued. A military study showed nearly a 20 percent decline in maximum muscle force after soldiers had completed a long overnight flight across multiple time zones. The fact is, even if you play a sport regularly, you're playing right up against the edge of injury unless you build substantial reserve strength. In tennis you're one late, hard shot away from a bad shoulder or tennis elbow. When hiking, you're one step away from twisting your knee. By reserves I mean the ability to produce sudden, rapid surges of power, between 50 percent and 100 percent more than you need to lift your body weight.

TEST YOURSELF

The following series of tests will help you determine if you have leg weakness. They measure the entire lower-extremity strength, not just the quadriceps. There is also a separate test for isolated strength of the quadriceps muscle. This is the most important muscle for the protection of the knee, but testing it requires sophisticated equipment, whereas testing overall leg strength can be done at home or at most local gyms or health clubs. Use these tests to follow your progress. Don't feel you have to do all the tests. If you're in good condition, you can skip the first couple. Of the remaining tests, pick one leg press or squat test and one knee extension test.

Testing at Home

Here's a graded testing program for you to do at home. If you're strong and athletic, you may want to skip straight to test 3. If you know you have some weakness, start with the two easier tests.

1. Getting up from a chair. Do you use your hands to assist you when rising from a deep-seated sofa or chair? Can your legs do it alone? If not, you don't have the most basic power required by your quadriceps. You should be able to lift your own body weight with ease. If you weigh 150 pounds, you need the squat strength of 150 pounds to get out of the chair easily. The more you weigh, the more strength you need both to protect the joint and for functional strength.

When walking down stairs, do you need to use a handrail? That's another tip-off that you may lack the basic strength you need to undertake daily activities of living.

2. Tape measure. Six inches above the middle of the kneecap, measure the diameter of each thigh. Compare the two readings. An inequality signals a loss of muscle mass and a loss of strength in the smaller thigh.

3. Squats. This is a simple yet highly effective way of testing leg strength. I like this test because squats are such an important part of training, so you can test and train with the same exercise. Determine the number of squats you can perform, bending your legs into a 90-degree angle, without using a wall for support.

Directions: Stand with your feet six inches apart. Squat until your thighs are parallel to the floor, but don't let your knees go in front of your ankles, then return to an upright position. Record the number of repetitions to a maximum of fifty. For more detailed instructions on squats, see Chapter 10.

Here are the numbers you should be able to do for your age. Since this study was done with adults over age thirty-four, there are no values for younger adults. You can extrapolate from the values in the table. For instance, a male thirty to thirty-four years of age should be able to do roughly forty-seven squats.

TABLE 4-1. SQUATS

Age	Males	Females
35–39	46	27
40–44	45	18
45–49	40	26
50–54	41	18

Source: H. Alaranta, H. Hurri, M. Heliovaara, A. Soukka, and R. Harju, "Non-dynamic Trunk Performance Tests: Reliability and Normative Data," *Scandinavian Journal of Rehabilitation Medicine* 26 (1994): 211–215.

Squats shouldn't be done if they increase your joint pain, as opposed to creating "muscle burn." If you cannot tolerate squats, leg presses are a reasonable substitute, but you'll have to go to a gym to do them. Leg presses almost mimic squats in terms of muscle activation but are easier on the joints as they are not a weight-bearing exercise. They target the quadriceps, the hamstrings, and the gluteus maximus. They are normally performed on a machine where the legs are pressed against a weighted platform. The leg press is a much simpler exercise and is sometimes preferred for beginners as an alternative to squats.

If you failed any of these three tests—you could not get out of a chair or walk down a flight of stairs unassisted, or have one quadriceps smaller than the other, or could not do the number of squats suggested in Table 4-1—you have substantial muscular weakness and are at significant risk of further wear and tear and injury to your joints. If you passed all three tests, you may still have significant muscle weakness, which can be revealed by the next step.

Testing at the Gym

As we've seen, there's no good way to quantitate testing at home where you can't get hard numbers on your absolute strength. Even the most modest gym should have the two machines required to measure your strength accurately. The first test, a leg press, is for overall leg strength, including your quads, buttocks muscles, hamstrings, and calf muscles. The second, a knee extension, is specific for quad strength.

1. Leg press. Here's an easy way to test your overall leg strength. Most gyms have a leg press machine. See what the maximum amount of weight is that you can lift on a single attempt. As a rough rule of thumb, you should be able to lift twice your weight. You'll see that the test scores allow for an age-related decline. For the purposes of this book, the goal is to close in on twice your weight regardless of age. Remember, as strength declines with aging, wear and tear on your joints increases.

These procedures were developed by the Cooper Institute for Aerobics Research using Universal's leg press machine.

1. Seat yourself in the chair with the ball of the foot on the crease of the pedal. Set the knee angle to 70 degrees if you have no knee pain or orthopedic problems. Otherwise, start with a smaller angle that you're comfortable with, as little as 30 degrees if you feel you're at risk of hurting yourself. Estimate how much weight you can lift in one maximal effort. If you're in decent shape, start with your body weight. Set the weight stack to your body weight. Do two to three repetitions and gauge how you feel.

2. Breathe out on exertion.

3. Progressively increase the resistance until you can no longer lift the weight stack. The first two or three trials serve as warm up lifts to prepare you for a maximal lift on the fifth or sixth trial. You can increase by 10-, 20-, 30-pound or more increments between trials to home in on the maximal amount you are capable of lifting. As you close in on your maximum, increase the weight stack in smaller increments.

4. Once you have achieved a maximal effort, take the number of pounds you lifted and divide it by your body weight.

5. Use the tables below to determine your fitness category. The numbers represent the number of times your body weight you can lift. The fittest people can lift more than twice their body weight.

TABLE 4-2. LEG PRESSES

Percentile	Age 20–29	Age 30–39	Age 40–49	Age 50–59	Age 60+
			Men		
90	2.27	2.07	1.92	1.80	1.73
80	2.13	1.93	1.82	1.71	1.62
70	2.05	1.85	1.74	1.64	1.56
60	1.97	1.77	1.68	1.58	1.49
50	1.91	1.71	1.62	1.52	1.43
40	1.83	1.65	1.57	1.46	1.38
30	1.74	1.59	1.51	1.39	1.30
20	1.63	1.52	1.44	1.32	1.25
10	1.51	1.43	1.35	1.22	1.16
			Women		
90	1.82	1.61	1.48	1.37	1.32
80	1.68	1.47	1.37	1.25	1.18
70	1.58	1.39	1.29	1.17	1.13
60	1.50	1.33	1.23	1.10	1.04
50	1.44	1.27	1.18	1.05	.99
40	1.37	1.21	1.13	.99	.93
30	1.27	1.15	1.08	.95	.88
20	1.22	1.09	1.02	.88	.85
10	1.14	1.00	.94	.78	.72

Source: *Physical Fitness Specialist Manual* (Dallas, Tex.: Cooper Institute, 2002). Reprinted with permission.

The one-rep-max test is only for the very fit. If you have had previous injuries, have demonstrated weakness on the home tests, or have arthritis, problems with your kneecaps, or other forms of joint damage, avoid the one-rep max.

2. Leg extension. The best way to test the quadriceps directly in the gym is on a leg extension machine as this is the only exercise that isolates the quadriceps. The general gold standard is the one-repetition maximum, the heaviest weight that can be lifted only once using good form. Here are the basic directions from the American College of Sports Medicine.

1. Perform a light warm-up of five to ten repetitions at 40 to 60 percent of the maximum you think you can lift.

2. Following a one-minute rest with light stretching, do three to five repetitions at 60 to 80 percent of what you think your maximum is.

3. You should now be closing in on your one-repetition maximum. Add a small amount of additional weight and try to lift the weight once. If the lift is successful, rest for three to five minutes. Then add another small amount of weight. Continue until you can no longer increase the weight.

4. The one-repetition maximum is reported as the weight of the last successfully completed lift.*

To score this test, take the maximum weight you were able to lift and divide it by your body weight. Look for that number in the left-hand column on the next page. Your score, from 1 to 10, appears in the right-hand column.

---

* American College of Sports Medicine, *Guidelines for Exercise Testing and Prescription,* 6th ed. (Baltimore, Md.: Lippincott, Williams & Wilkins, 2000).

TABLE 4-3. LEG EXTENSION STRENGTH-TO-BODY-WEIGHT RATIO

Men	Points
.80	10
.75	9
.70	8
.65	7
.60	6
.55	5
.50	4
.45	3
.40	2
.35	1

Women	Points
.70	10
.65	9
.60	8
.55	7
.52	6
.50	5
.45	4
.40	3
.35	2
.30	1

Score: 9–10: excellent; 7–8: good; 5–6: average; 3–4: fair; 1–2: poor.

Source: Vivian H. Heyward, *Advanced Fitness Assessment and Exercise Prescription,* 3rd ed. (Champaign, Ill.: Human Kinetics, 1998).

These norms apply only to college-aged men and women. To date, there are no published leg extension strength norms for middle-aged or older adults.

Attempting a one-repetition maximum with heavy weights can place an undue and unreasonable amount of stress on the muscles, bones, and connective tissues. Kevin Wilk, a world-renowned physical therapist who is currently the national director of research and education for HealthSouth Rehabilitation in Birmingham, Alabama, is comfortable with patients who have mild to moderate osteoarthritis using the one-repetition maximum as long as they have a good warm-up. However, beware of joint pain, bone pain along the medial or lateral joint line, and pain underneath the kneecap, which should be a signal to stop. Even mild joint pain means that you should lighten the load, change the exercise, or take a day or two off. Mild to moderate muscle soreness is acceptable, says Wilk, but be careful not to strain your muscles.

Professional Testing by a Physical Therapist

The Isokinetic Test The gold-standard test for quad strength is the isokinetic test. Here's why. With the leg extension performed in the gym, you're limited by your weakest link. Let's say your weak spot is when your knee is extended to 45 degrees. You'll never know how strong you are at, say, 30 degrees and 90 degrees because the weakness at the 45-degree angle limits the amount of weight you can use.

An isokinetic test can give you the most specific information about strength, including absolute values throughout the full range of movement. In other words, you can get a measure of maximal muscle contraction at every joint angle. This test requires very sophisticated and expensive machinery such as Cybex or Biodex. The only drawback is the availability of the equipment and the need for a skilled clinician to assess the test. The advantage is that you'll find weaknesses you wouldn't find any other way. This is especially important if you have had a minor knee injury in your past. Kevin Wilk looked at people who performed normally on a manual strength test and found that they had equal strength in both legs. The isokinetic test, however, showed that one leg was 28 percent weaker than the other.

In fact, Dr. Michael Hurley reports that even ten years after an injury to their knee, people who believe they have gotten over it quite well and report no functional problems will find they suffer from weakness they aren't aware of.

What to Expect You'll be asked to extend and flex your knee. The principle of the isokinetic device is that the operator can choose a specific speed for your test. No matter how hard you work your muscles, you will not be able to exceed that speed limit. The tester will typically test you at several different speed settings. This allows the physical therapist to determine where in your joint range of motion you are weak and at what speed. For instance, weakness may be detected at the 40-degree angle at slow speeds. The physical therapist can then give you a precise prescription. The beauty of the test is that it isolates the knee so you are looking purely at the function of your quadriceps and hamstring without interference from other joints or muscles. Since it's easy to disguise knee weakness by using other joints and muscles, isokinetic testing is the only sure way to determine the weakness of the muscles critical to the knee. Also, since you're pressing against hydraulic fluid and not a real weight, there's much less likelihood that you will injure yourself. If you have a known injury or arthritis, I'd recommend using training devices that work on this hydraulic principle so that you minimize the chance of being hurt in testing and maximize the chance of getting a good result.

Solutions Weakness of the quadriceps muscle is common in patients with wear and tear. It is clear that strengthening the quadriceps can help: according to the National Institutes of Health, a relatively small increase in strength (20 percent for men and 25 percent for women) can lead to a 20 to 30 percent decrease in risk of wear-and-tear arthritis. We'll look at how to build strength in the chapter on building muscular strength. If you've done poorly on these tests, be assured that there is a lot you can do quickly to become much stronger to protect your joints and live a healthier, better life.

5

Overload

Two hundred ten miserable pounds, ugh! It was the heaviest I'd ever been—a good twenty pounds over my regular weight, but then that's what happens with wear and tear. Everything hurt: my knees, my hips, my shoulders. The more pain, the less activity I engaged in, and the pounds just kept piling on. I'd always heard that weight loss leads to a decrease in arthritis pain, but boy, can weight gain ever increase the pain! How to get it off? The biggest problem is that painful joints make your best weapon, vigorous physical activity, tough to follow through on at best. The decrease in your ability to exercise without pain often results in even greater weight gain. What's more, too much weight can be extremely destructive.

The Baptist College of Health Sciences in Memphis has one of the finest health care educational programs in the South. On a recent visit there I got to talking about arthritis. Doctors and professors described a phenomenon that made my jaw drop: obese women were destroying their knees, blowing them out with such severity, that the only therapeutic choice was amputation. These women developed weakness of their quads, limited range of motion, and arthritis. Now add to that the exceptionally heavy heel strike we saw in Chapter 1, and you can begin to imagine the destructive forces. Although these women are the extreme, every little bit of extra weight hurts. And women with excess pounds may often have the fatal combination of quad weakness and heavy heel strike. The risk of knee arthritis is significantly increased among patients with more excess weight, and these poor women paid the price.

The conventional wisdom: A few extra pounds isn't a big deal.
The real deal: Lose the weight, lose the pain.

Wear and tear is accelerating at a ferocious rate. Little wonder! A recent Rand study showed that 36 percent of adults are overweight and another 23 percent are obese. The same study showed that obesity is associated with more chronic conditions and worse physical health–related quality of life than smoking or drinking! And one of those conditions is arthritis!

Why? Boston University's Dr. Felson explains, "Increased force across the weight-bearing joints probably explains most of the risk."

TEST: ARE YOU THE RIGHT WEIGHT?

Use the following table to determine whether you are the appropriate weight.

Here's how the table works. Find your height in inches in the left-hand column. Then follow across the row until you find your present weight. Now go up that column to the column head and read your BMI.

The National Heart, Lung, and Blood Institute has proposed that "doctors use body mass index (BMI) to assess patients because the index is simple, correlates to fatness, and applies to both men and women. A BMI of 25 to 29.9 is considered overweight and one 30 or above is considered obese."

TABLE 4-4. BODY MASS INDEX

BMI	19	20	21	22	23	24	25	26	27	28	29	30	31	32	33	34	35
Height (inches)								Body Weight (pounds)									
58	91	96	100	105	110	115	119	124	129	134	138	143	148	153	158	162	167
59	94	99	104	109	114	119	124	128	133	138	143	148	153	158	163	168	173
60	97	102	107	112	118	123	128	133	138	143	148	153	158	163	168	174	179
61	100	106	111	116	122	127	132	137	143	148	153	158	164	169	174	180	185
62	104	109	115	120	126	131	136	142	147	153	158	164	169	175	180	186	191
63	107	113	118	124	130	135	141	146	152	158	163	169	175	180	186	191	197
64	110	116	122	128	134	140	145	151	157	163	169	174	180	186	192	197	204
65	114	120	126	132	138	144	150	156	162	168	174	180	186	192	198	204	210
66	118	124	130	136	142	148	155	161	167	173	179	186	192	198	204	210	216
67	121	127	134	140	146	153	159	166	172	178	185	191	198	204	211	217	223
68	125	131	138	144	151	158	164	171	177	184	190	197	203	210	216	223	230
69	128	135	142	149	155	162	169	176	182	189	196	203	209	216	223	230	236
70	132	139	146	153	160	167	174	181	188	195	202	209	216	222	229	236	243
71	136	143	150	157	165	172	179	186	193	200	208	215	222	229	236	243	250
72	140	147	154	162	169	177	184	191	199	206	213	221	228	235	242	250	258
73	144	151	159	166	174	182	189	197	204	212	219	227	235	242	250	257	265
74	148	155	163	171	179	186	194	202	210	218	225	233	241	249	256	264	272
75	152	160	168	176	184	192	200	208	216	224	232	240	248	256	264	272	279
76	156	164	172	180	189	197	205	213	221	230	238	246	254	263	271	279	287

TABLE 4-5. BODY MASS INDEX

BMI	36	37	38	39	40	41	42	43	44	45	46	47	48	49	50	51	52	53	54
Height (inches)									Body Weight (pounds)										
58	172	177	181	186	191	196	201	205	210	215	220	224	229	234	239	244	248	253	258
59	178	183	188	193	198	203	208	212	217	222	227	232	237	242	247	252	257	262	267
60	184	189	194	199	204	209	215	220	225	230	235	240	245	250	255	261	266	271	276
61	190	195	201	206	211	217	222	227	232	238	243	248	254	259	264	269	275	280	285
62	196	202	207	213	218	224	229	235	240	246	251	256	262	267	273	278	284	289	295
63	203	208	214	220	225	231	237	242	248	254	259	265	270	278	282	287	293	299	304
64	209	215	221	227	232	238	244	250	256	262	267	273	279	285	291	296	302	308	314
65	216	222	228	234	240	246	252	258	264	270	276	282	288	294	300	306	312	318	324
66	223	229	235	241	247	253	260	266	272	278	284	291	297	303	309	315	322	328	334
67	230	236	242	249	255	261	268	274	280	287	293	299	306	312	319	325	331	338	344
68	236	243	249	256	262	269	276	282	289	295	302	308	315	322	328	335	341	348	354
69	243	250	257	263	270	277	284	291	297	304	311	318	324	331	338	345	351	358	365
70	250	257	264	271	278	285	292	299	306	313	320	327	334	341	348	355	362	369	376
71	257	265	272	279	286	293	301	308	315	322	329	338	343	351	358	365	372	379	386
72	265	272	279	287	294	302	309	316	324	331	338	346	353	361	368	375	383	390	397
73	272	280	288	295	302	310	318	325	333	340	348	355	363	371	378	386	393	401	408
74	280	287	295	303	311	319	326	334	342	350	358	365	373	381	389	396	404	412	420
75	287	295	303	311	319	327	335	343	351	359	367	375	383	391	399	407	415	423	431
76	295	304	312	320	328	336	344	353	361	369	377	385	394	402	410	418	426	435	443

What can you do now? With dozens of different diet plans and hundreds of different books about weight loss, what's the best approach? The answers are in Chapter 12, "Lighten the Load."

PART TWO

Solutions: Beating Wear and Tear

6

Kill the Pain

Sunday mornings in the winter are D day for Dad! The morning begins at the bottom of Mount Mansfield's high-speed quad ski lift. The best and fastest racers are in line at 7:30. After several hours of trying to follow their arcing Super G turns down the fast, steep, sometimes icy slopes, it's time for tennis—to be precise, two hours of retribution at the hands of my fourteen-year-old son on the tennis court. His lightning-fast returns send poor old Dad running for shots he wouldn't have had a prayer of getting even twenty years ago. At 3:30 it's time for a punishing twenty-kilometer ski up to the Trapp Family lodge over the most demanding terrain in the eastern United States. Quite a day! But by nightfall my muscles and joints are crying out in agony: Advil, Advil, Advil! I could hardly wait to start gulping those little brown pills—Father's little helpers—much like the fifties-style adman eyeing his first martini. Within an hour, glorious relief. Wow. Had I ever felt better! No question about it, pain relievers work wonders—and quickly. There's a real place for them, but consumers beware! Pain medications taken in high doses over weeks or months can have serious side effects. While I'm one of the first to advocate fast, powerful pain relief, there is also a second objective: safety.

The **conventional wisdom:** Painkillers let you move your joints more freely.

The **real deal:** Kill your pain, but be judicious.

Let's take a look at the available options.

THE FIRST LINE OF DEFENSE

Acetaminophen

Brand Name: Tylenol Tylenol? Kid's stuff, you may say. "Too weak, too watered down" is the usual attitude. Weekend warriors often ignore acetaminophen and jump right to the full-strength stuff, but that could be a mistake.

The American College of Rheumatology (ACR) recommends acetaminophen as first-line drug therapy for patients with mild to moderate pain from knee osteoarthritis. This is the first choice of many rheumatologists because of its low-side-effect profile. Simply put, it's not going to burn a hole through your stomach. Acetaminophen has been found effective in alleviating pain in patients with osteoarthritis in a placebo-controlled trial and when compared to other pain relievers.

As much as you may lust for stronger pain relievers, the experts all say acetaminophen merits a trial as initial therapy in patients with mild to moderate pain. There is also evidence that acetaminophen is underdosed. Forty-one percent of women "with severe lower limb OA pain" were using less than 20 percent of the recommended maximum dose.

How Well Does it Work? In one study, 184 patients with osteoarthritic knee pain were randomized to receive acetaminophen (4,000 milligrams daily) or ibuprofen (1,200 or 2,400 milligrams daily) for four weeks. Among patients with low and medium baseline pain scores, the two drugs performed similarly. In the highest pain group, high-dose ibuprofen worked only marginally better than acetaminophen. That's pretty surprising when you consider the weakling image of acetaminophen! Acetaminophen is a pure pain reliever and has no anti-inflammatory effect.

Use For mild to moderate arthritis.

Safety Up to a total of 4 grams in three or four doses a day is considered safe. As with any other drug, this is one you do not want to gulp down in handfuls.

It's *not* as safe as water, which is the way many people consume it. In rare circumstances, an overdosage can lead to liver failure. The risk is especially high if you consume alcohol. That's not meant to frighten you. Stay within the safe limits, and you'll be fine. The safe limit is printed on the package insert. To be clear, here it is: Maximum dose not to exceed 4 grams per day. If you consume three or more drinks a day, the FDA recommends consulting your physician.

However, acetaminophen is considered the safest of the over-the-counter pain relievers.

Anthony R. Temple, M.D., vice president of medical and regulatory science for the McNeil Consumer & Specialty Pharmaceuticals Division of McNeil-PPC, Inc., takes issue with the ACR guideline that patients with chronic alcohol abuse should avoid taking acetaminophen, citing research that demonstrates that the product is safe, even for alcoholics in an acute detoxification setting.

The renewed warnings were sparked by a report from the University of Texas Southwestern Medical Center. Researchers tracked more than three hundred cases of acute liver failure at twenty-two hospitals and found that 38 percent of them were associated with excessive acetaminophen use. What surprised the researchers were not the findings as much as the ignorance among other physicians. In a recent survey, just under half knew that most cases of liver toxicity from acetaminophen result from overdoses. A common mistake is mixing alcohol with acetaminophen; alcohol hampers the liver's ability to clear toxins from the blood and can lead to an overdose.

Be careful not to inadvertently overdose by taking cold or flu remedies at the same time. Many contain acetaminophen, which means that if you're already taking 4 grams of Tylenol, you'll be over the limit if you're also taking cold and flu medications containing it. Still, most reported cases of acetaminophen toxicity occur when people take two to three times the suggested dose in a 24 to 48-hour period. Dr. William Lee, one of the study's leaders, admits that even though it's a bit cautious, it may be better to recommend a maximum of 2 grams of acetaminophen to be safe.

Other Warnings

Prolongs bleeding times: If you're taking a blood thinner, be aware that acetaminophen prolongs the half-life of warfarin sodium (Coumadin). If you begin acetaminophen treatment, you'll want to make sure your doctor measures your prothrombin time more often.

However, most doctors recommend acetaminophen for people who are on blood thinners because it still has a higher safety profile then many other pain relievers.

Acetaminophen with codeine

For more powerful pain relief combined with the safety of acetaminophen, consider adding codeine. Product names include Fioricet, Phenaphen with Codeine, and Tylenol with Codeine.

Tylenol Arthritis Pain

This helps relieve osteoarthritis and joint-related pain with time-release caplets. The caplets have a patented bilayer. The first layer dissolves immediately to give you immediate relief, while the second layer is time-released to give you up to eight hours of pain relief so you can take them less frequently. In addition, the dosage is 650 milligrams (mg) and differs from regular Tylenol, which is 325 milligrams.

Side Effects Constipation, dizziness, light-headedness, drowsiness, nausea, tiredness, weakness, or vomiting.

Other Products

For very severe pain, your doctor may consider Darvon or Ultram.

THE NEXT STEP

NSAIDs

Brand Names: Advil, Motrin, Nuprin Nonsteroidal anti-inflammatory drugs (NSAIDs) are among the most commonly used drugs for osteoarthritis. NSAIDs have the ability to reduce inflammation and pain by blocking the action of certain body chemicals called prostaglandins, which play a role in causing inflammation and pain.

These are what most of us think of when we go for full-strength over-the-counter pain relief: ibuprofen. Ibuprofen is powerful, effective, and quick. It's the drug of choice for patients with severe arthritis and the second choice of patients with mild to moderate arthritis after they've failed a course of acetaminophen.

Use For mild to moderate arthritis.

Dosage Milder NSAIDs such as Advil and Motrin are available over the counter. These medications should not be taken for more than ten days without a doctor's visit. More powerful NSAIDs require a prescription.

People Who Should Avoid Ibuprofen Some people should not take ibuprofen. These include:

◆ People with a history of asthma attacks, hives, or other allergic reactions to aspirin or other NSAIDs.

◆ People with peptic ulcer disease.

◆ People with poor kidney function. If you start talking about taking higher doses than recommended for over-the-counter drugs, there are a whole host of other side effects. The most notable is adverse renal function. The National Kidney Foundation has taken a position urging caution in the use of NSAIDs by patients with kidney disease. Instead, it recommends acetaminophen for those patients.

◆ People taking blood-thinning medications (anticoagulants), such as Coumadin. Because of an increased risk of bleeding, their blood-clotting times should be monitored carefully.

◆ Patients taking lithium, who may develop toxic blood lithium levels.

◆ Patients undergoing surgery. Ibuprofen should be discontinued at least two days in advance of surgery because of mild interference with clotting.

Side Effects Abdominal pain, dizziness, drowsiness, fluid retention, heartburn, indigestion, light-headedness, nausea, nightmares, rash, and changes in liver function tests. Ibuprofen should be taken with meals.

Warnings You may think the following warnings are a bit overdone, but if you take medication day in, day out, you'll want to know.

Bleeding: The greatest hazard of ibuprofen is that of bleeding from the stomach or a part of the small intestine called the duodenum. The duodenum is the first portion of the small intestine into which the contents of the stomach empties. It's the most common site of ulcers.

Data from epidemiologic studies show that among persons sixty-five years or older, "20 to 30 percent of all hospitalizations and deaths due to peptic ulcer disease are attributable to therapy with NSAIDs." In the elderly, the risk of a catastrophic bleed is dose-dependent: the more you take, the higher the risk. Every year, 16,500 NSAID-related deaths occur among patients with rheumatoid arthritis or wear-and-tear arthritis in the United States.

Alcohol Warning: When used with NSAIDs, alcohol can cause stomach bleeding. If you drink more than three alcoholic beverages per day, you're at increased risk of developing stomach ulcers when taking ibuprofen.

Comparing Risks More people die each year from the toxic ef-

fects of NSAIDs than from liver toxicity caused by acetaminophen. On balance, if you take the recommended dose of acetaminophen, your risk of developing serious complications is extremely
small.

How can you get the pain-relieving ability of ibuprofen without such a big risk of bleeding? There are two ways. First, consider
taking drugs called COX-2 inhibitors (see below). Second, consider
taking drugs that cut the risk of bleeding.

Aspirin

Aspirin is a major pain reliever used for rheumatoid arthritis
but not for wear-and-tear arthritis. Dr. Marc C. Hochberg, a leading arthritis researcher and head of the Division of Rheumatology
at the University of Maryland, states, "Aspirin is no longer used to
any great degree for treatment of OA. This is because of the short
half-life and requirement for high doses that have a high frequency
of side effects."

COX-2 Inhibitors

COX-2 inhibitors have become the latest rage in arthritis medications. Simply put, COX-2 inhibitors are a safer version of
ibuprofen and are prescribed as an alternative. Here's why. Ibuprofen, like all NSAIDs, inhibits two critical substances in your body,
COX-1 *and* COX-2. When COX-2 is inhibited, your pain is relieved and inflammation reduced. Inhibiting COX-1 strips away
some of the stomach's ability to protect itself from bleeding. By
eliminating the COX-1 inhibitor from NSAIDs, scientists were able
to develop drugs that retain the arthritis-pain-relieving properties
but decrease the risk of bleeding from the stomach and duodenum.

Thus, the chief selling point of COX-2 inhibitors is that they
produce significantly fewer stomach problems including bleeding
ulcers. There are two popular brands. The first COX-2 inhibitor
was Celebrex. The second to hit the market was Vioxx. There is
also a third called Bextra.

When researchers examine the stomach by viewing it with

an endoscope, they have demonstrated that these two COX-2 inhibitors are associated with fewer ulcers than comparable NSAIDs and a similar rate to that of a placebo. Several studies have been published, in particular the VIGOR (Vioxx Gastrointestinal Outcomes Research) and the CLASS (Celecoxib Long-term Arthritis Safety Study), which have shown a clear reduction in serious gastrointestinal side effects, including ulcers, bleeding, and obstruction. However, these products are no more effective than existing NSAIDs.

Doctors worry that advertising campaigns may lead patients to ask for COX-2 inhibitors as drugs of first choice, skipping over acetaminophen and over-the-counter NSAIDs, such as ibuprofen, which may be equally effective for mild to moderate disease. However, for severe disease and moderate to severe pain, some physicians feel they can give patients far higher doses of COX-2 inhibitors than of ibuprofen to gain greater control over the pain.

If pain keeps you from engaging in any activities and other pain relievers aren't working, you might consider the COX-2 inhibitors, especially if you are at high risk of bleeding from your stomach.

Brand Name: Celebrex Celebrex was approved on December 31, 1998, by the Food and Drug Administration to treat the signs and symptoms of both osteoarthritis and adult rheumatoid arthritis (RA). Celebrex is also approved as a possible preventive agent for patients at high risk of colon cancer due to a rare and devastating genetic disease called familial adenomatous polyposis. Celebrex improved patients' ability to perform daily activities, such as dressing, walking, and going up or down stairs. There were up to 85 percent fewer ulcers seen on visual examination of the stomach when compared to naproxen, a nonselective NSAID, after twelve weeks of use. If you're taking aspirin therapy to prevent a heart attack, you can combine that therapy with Celebrex. The increased risk of stomach ulcers with combined ASA (acetylsalicylic acid, or aspirin) and Celebrex is not known.

Dosage: The recommended therapeutic dosage for osteoarthritis is 200 milligrams daily. Once-a-day and twice-a-day dosing regimens are equally effective in providing sustained relief. Celebrex is available in 100- and 200-milligram capsules.

Brand Name: Vioxx This was the second COX-2 to be approved. Vioxx resulted in significantly fewer clinically important "events" such as bleeding stomach ulcers than did treatment with naproxen. The two drugs had similar rates of clinical effectiveness.

Dosage: The recommended starting dose of Vioxx is 12.5 milligrams once daily. Some patients may receive additional benefit by increasing the dose to 25 milligrams once daily. The maximum recommended daily dose is 25 milligrams.

Warnings Patients with high blood pressure, congestive heart failure, or mild to moderate renal failure should be cautious about taking COX-2 inhibitors as well as NSAIDs. Patients with a history of allergic reactions to sulfonamide should not take Celebrex.

A recent study reported by University of Pennsylvania researchers in the *Science Journal* suggests that COX-2 inhibitors may increase the risk of heart attacks in people with heart disease. This study reinforces an earlier study that found a group of Vioxx users to suffer twice the risk of heart attacks as users of an older painkiller. There is still much research that needs to be done to determine this risk, as this recent study's subjects were mice. Eric Topol of the Cleveland Clinic states, "Now the only thing we're really missing is quantifying the magnitude of the risk." He warns that in the meantime, people with heart disease should be cautious when taking COX-2 inhibitors because there could be some risk.

Brand Name: Bextra This is the latest COX-2 inhibitor to hit the market. Several clinical studies have shown that a single 10-milligram tablet of Bextra is just as effective in relieving arthritis pain as two 500-milligram tablets of naproxen, a common arthritis pain reliever.

Dosage: The recommended dose of Bextra is one 10-milligram tablet daily.

Cotherapy

We've seen the significant long-term risk of developing bleeding from the stomach if you use certain pain relievers on a daily basis. There is another strategy, one that I myself use and recommend. It's called "cotherapy," which means taking a second drug whose sole function is to protect your stomach and duodenum from bleeding.

How well do they work? In a study of 8,843 patients with severe arthritis, 200 milligrams of Cytotec (misoprostol) four times a day reduced the incidence of complicated ulcers, including those with perforation, bleeding, and obstruction, by 51 percent (63). Cytotec is a synthetic prostaglandin that works by replacing the prostaglandin stripped away by NSAIDs.

Brand Names: Prilosec, Prevacid Prilosec (omeprazole) and Prevacid (lansoprazole) are as effective as misoprostol at treating ulcers. They also reduce the upset stomach or dyspepsia from NSAIDs. Although not approved by the FDA for use in prophylaxis, they are being widely used for this purpose. One popular combination is Prilosec and Motrin. There is one drug that combines the NSAID diclofenac sodium with misoprostol. Marketed under the name Arthrotec, the drug is available only by prescription. H2 blockers or H2 antagonists stop the stomach from producing as much acid. H2 blockers may be used to treat ulcers as well but have not been found to be as effective as misoprostol. H2 blockers include such drugs as Tagamet (cimetidine), Zantac (ranitidine hydrochloride), Pepcid (famotidine), and Axid Pulvules (nizatidine). There is one theoretical concern with H2 blockers: one study indicated that they might mask the early symptoms of stomach ulcers.

The downside of cotherapy is that you are adding another medication and thus running the risk of a drug interaction. Since you'll need a prescription for most of these, you'll want to discuss the pros and cons of using cotherapy versus a COX-2 inhibitor to reduce your pain. Medications are not the only way to relieve pain. You may also want to consider the use of local anesthetics, injections, or acupuncture as well as the nonpharmaceutical approaches described in this book.

Tramadol

Tramadol hydrochloride is a nonnarcotic analgesic used to treat severe chronic pain. Tramadol probably works better than acetaminophen. However, there is a new version called Ultracet, a combination of tramadol and acetaminophen, that clearly works better than acetaminophen alone. The FDA recently approved it. Tramadol has the advantage of having a slightly different mechanism than acetaminophen even though they are both centrally active. They seem to work in different areas of the brain so you get additional pain relief. The tramadol relieves pain by binding to certain receptors called *mu*-opioid receptors in the central nervous system. Tramadol also inhibits the reuptake of norepinephrine and serotonin, which may elicit the pain relief. Tramadol does have an opioid pharmacology, but it's a little different. Although opioids have tolerance and dependence problems, tramadol does not appear to. However, tramadol may cause dizziness, somnolence, nausea, constipation, sweating, and pruritus similar to those of other opioids.

Opioids

The new American Pain Society guidelines for the management of osteoarthritis emphasize the importance of opioids for severe pain. You may want to consider these with your physician if you do have severe pain and other measures have failed.

OTHER REMEDIES

Topical Analgesics

Here is a unique way to reduce the amount of medication you take orally: use a topical analgesic preparation such as Zostrix or Capzasin-P. They can be quite effective while helping you decrease or stop taking oral medications. Their scientific underpinning is their ability to stimulate or irritate the nerve endings, distracting the brain's attention from musculoskeletal pain. For this reason they are called counterirritants. Dr. Anthony Temple says that they are absorbed into the superficial tissues of the skin; they irritate the nerve endings and provide a local irritating, burning sensation. When that is transmitted back to the spinal column, it overrides the pain sensation from the related joint. If you have pain in a couple of small joints, then topical analgesics work great. But if you have pretty severe knee osteoarthritis, you're probably not going to get significant relief.

Methylsalicylate Creams These work by stimulating or irritating the nerve endings. Brand names include Ben-Gay, Flex-all, Mobisyl, and Sportscreme. Don't use these if you are allergic to aspirin.

Capsaicin Cream An ingredient found in cayenne peppers is the foundation of capsaicin. Despite its low-tech base, it has a high-tech mechanism of action. The cream works by depleting a neurotransmitter called "substance P," which may send pain messages to the brain. Products including capsaicin are Zostrix, Zostrix-HP, Capzaicin-P, and Menthacin. Capsaicin cream is probably the most effective counterirritant.

Topical creams have two huge advantages over medications taken by mouth. First, there isn't the risk of kidney or liver damage or of bleeding. Second, they don't appear to interfere with repair of the joints. For those reasons they are worth a try. You can start using topical analgesics even while you're taking other medications. Studies have shown you can reduce your dependence on NSAIDs.

Capsaicin cream should be applied to the symptomatic joint four times daily. You may notice some burning or stinging for the first several days you use it, but that will fade with time. It is also important to wash your hands after using capsaicin cream and to avoid getting it into your eyes.

Injections

These are alternatives to oral medications, which don't have risks to internal organs such as the stomach, kidney, or liver.

Hyaluronic Acid

Use: For mild to moderate knee osteoarthritis.

Called "viscosupplements," these products are injected directly into the joint to replace hyaluronic acid. Hyaluronic acid gives joint fluid its viscosity, which acts to dampen shock. However, hyaluronic acid appears to break down in arthritic joints. The FDA has approved two preparations of hyaluronan. The approval is specifically for the treatment of wear-and-tear knee arthritis when patients have not responded to nondrug therapy and acetaminophen. To date, differences in clinical effectiveness between these preparations have not been demonstrated. Originally, doctors thought that this was a joint replacement fluid that acted as a shock absorber. Now they're not so sure. Since the benefit lasts longer than the time supplements remain in the knee, their mechanism of action is unclear. One theory is that they inhibit the toxic soup of chemicals that destroy the joint. Those include cytokines and prostaglandins. Hyaluronic acid may also stimulate the production of cartilage and slow its destruction. Whether this provides an additional benefit is being studied. Some advocates believe that hyaluronic acid therapy may slow the progression of cartilage damage. How well does hyaluronic acid work for pain? The pain relief may be slower in onset than that brought about by steroids, but the effect is considerably longer with hyaluronan injections.

Dr. Vijay Vad, a sports medicine specialist at the Hospital for Special Surgery in New York City, has seen tremendous results using hylan (a hyaluronic acid product). "If you have failed other forms of conservative treatments, then hylan therapy may be a good option in the well-selected patients." This is because hylan is more invasive and expensive: thus its use is reserved for people who have failed other treatments such as NSAIDs, physical therapy, and cortisone injection. Dr. Vad has seen tremendous results using hylan in patients who have mild to moderate arthritis on X rays and still have significant muscle strength. However, he states that the effectiveness of hylan is greatest when combined with other modalities. "Hylan's effectiveness is maximized by good patient selection, which is either Grade Three or less OA, and when it's combined with a joint lavage (flushing the joint) prior to instillation of the hylan, combined with a precise rehabilitation program." Dr. Vad also runs one of the few programs in the country that injects hyaluronic acid into the hip. He first washes out the arthritic debris in the joint, then injects the hyaluronic acid. The results to date have been quite encouraging, he reports.

If you can't take NSAIDs, have experienced adverse effects, or have not been helped by them, these products may be just what you're looking for. The downsides? You may notice pain at the injection site. Some patients also note joint pain and swelling after the injection.

Dosage:

- **Hyaluronate (Hyalgan):** Five 2-milliliter injections once a week for five weeks.
- **Hylan G-F 20 (Synvisc):** Three 2-milliliter injections over fifteen days.

Side Effects: Swelling, heat, and redness at injection site. Pain and fluid collection around the site. Allergic reaction is possible if the patient is allergic to avian proteins, bird feathers, or eggs.

Steroids For quick, temporary relief without major side effects, your doctor may elect to inject your joint with a steroid known as a glucocorticoid. Steroids are of greatest value if you have a painful swollen joint. Do steroids help or hinder the progression of your disease? That's an open question since they have a mix of both positive and negative effects on joint destruction. For example, while steroids may reduce levels of toxic chemicals such as cytokines, they also suppress the synthesis of key components of cartilage.

Dosage: 40 milligrams triamcinolone hexacetonide.

Many patients worry about the risk of joint infection with frequent injections, but the risk is exceedingly low if standard aseptic technique is used. Patients may experience mild flares of pain in the lining of the joint called the synovium. However, these flares are temporary and can be treated with pain medications and cold compresses as necessary.

Acupuncture

The National Institutes of Health is supporting research to evaluate "alternative treatments."

One such project, led by Dr. Brian M. Berman of the University of Maryland School of Medicine, evaluated seventy-three people with moderate to severe wear-and-tear arthritis of the knee that "could not be relieved by standard anti-inflammatory drugs." The patients were randomly assigned to either continue on anti-inflammatory drugs alone or to add eight weeks of acupuncture treatment. After three months, Berman reported that "acupuncture did reduce their pain, they had less stiffness, and they were able to function better."

Massage

Massage therapy is another form of alternative treatment that has also been found to be helpful. The American Massage Therapy Association claims that "research shows [that massage] reduces the heart rate, lowers blood pressure, increases blood circulation, relaxes muscles, improves range of motion, and increases endorphins, the body's natural painkillers. Therapeutic massage enhances medical treatment and helps people feel less anxious and stressed, relaxed yet more alert." Massage elicits pain relief by reducing muscle spasms and pain around an arthritic joint, relaxing stiff muscles and reducing swelling that accompanies arthritis. Massage therapy has also been utilized with hot and cold modalities such as ice packs or heating pads.

Insurance companies are adding therapies such as massage therapy and acupuncture to their policies.

Judy Piette, a physical therapist in Stockbridge, Georgia, adds, "I recommend that people not use massage over a joint that is acutely inflamed—red, swollen, and tender. In that situation, I would apply ice to it for a few days to reduce the pain and swelling. Once the inflammation has calmed, a massage using large strokes is helpful. A deeper kneading-type massage can relax muscles and ease spasms. Massage therapy will not ease pain from swollen or inflamed joints."

Supplements

These naturally occurring substances are gaining favor even among traditional doctors. We'll look at one of them in this chapter and the others in the following chapter. The Arthritis Foundation has undertaken a very careful review of all available supplements. For each supplement reviewed here, I'll include their recommendation or lack thereof.

SAM-e *SAM*-e, short for S-adenosylmethionine, is touted as an effective way to treat the joint pain, stiffness, and inflammation of arthritis. There are several human studies showing that SAM-e relieves the pain of osteoarthritis as well as NSAIDs do. You may also notice a secondary benefit: psychopharmacologists such as Columbia University's Dr. Richard Brown use SAM-e as a first-line drug of choice for depression.

Many people who develop wear-and-tear arthritis become depressed by their pain and disability. You may want to discuss with your physician if SAM-e is an appropriate strategy for you to relieve joint pain and boost your mood. However, the reason the Arthritis Foundation does not recommend SAM-e is that it doesn't believe there is enough evidence to suggest that SAM-e works with arthritis.

Product Quality: SAM-e got an undeserved bad rap in the psychiatric community for its lack of effectiveness. On reanalyzing their data, doctors found that many patients were receiving low-grade, highly ineffective SAM-e that soured the results.

The brand you buy is critical. Early studies on the drug were flawed because patients took products that did not contain enough SAM-e. In January 2000 ConsumerLab.com purchased a total of thirteen brands of SAM-e products and then tested them to determine whether they possessed the labeled amounts of SAM-e. Over-all, nearly half (six out of thirteen) of the products did not pass test-ing. Among those not passing, the amount of SAM-e was, on average, less than half of the amount declared on the labels. In one product, the amount of SAM-e was below detectable levels (less than 5 percent of the labeled amount). Here are some of the pro-ducts that did pass ConsumerLab.com's test.

◆ Nature Made Joint Action 200 mg (1, 4-butanedisulfonate) Bonus note: This product also contains 500 mg glucosamine hydrochloride.
◆ NutraLife SAM-e 200 mg (tosylate disulphate)
◆ Puritan's Pride Inspired by Nature SAM-e 200 mg (form not indicated)
◆ Twinlab SAM-e, 200 mg (tosylate)

For more product reviews, you can log on to ConsumerLab.com's Web site, www.consumerlab.com.

Dosage: The generally recommended daily dose of SAM-e can range from 200 to 800 milligrams. Start with a dose of only 200 or 400 milligrams of SAM-e for the first day of therapy and increase it thereafter. These daily amounts should not be taken at once but in divided doses. For example, take 400 milligrams as 200 milligrams twice a day. If you're taking total of 800 milligrams a day, take 200 milligrams four times a day. Improvements can take from a few days to four or five weeks.

Side Effects: SAM-e may occasionally cause nausea and stom-ach upset, which may be reduced by taking enteric-coated prod-ucts, reducing the dosage, and taking it with meals.

Warnings: Individuals with manic-depressive illness should be aware that SAM-e could trigger a manic phase.

Consumers should check with a health care professional for a proper diagnosis before using dietary supplements and, due to po-tential drug interactions, should inform their health care providers of the dietary supplements they take. This may seem like an idle piece of bureaucracy, but internists and cardiologists are terrified by the interactions they see between dietary supplements and prescription medications, especially the tendency of some to increase bleeding times. While SAM-e poses little risk, herbal supplements in particular can be hazardous if taken with prescription drugs.

HOW PAIN RELIEVERS MAY INTERFERE WITH HEALING

In a study by Rush-Presbyterian-St. Luke's Medical Center, fifty-three subjects with symptomatic radiographic evidence of wear-and-tear arthritis of the knee were studied. When some of the subjects took acetaminophen, their pain was relieved. Seemed like a great idea. But when their gait was analyzed, those with the decreased pain tended to increase the load on the degenerated portion of their knee. Simply put, they loaded the worn-and-torn cartilage with forces high enough to do further damage to the joint.

We know that the knee joint can move from side to side as you walk. When it moves to the inside, it is called "adduction." Imagine that as your heel strikes the ground, your knee bows slightly to the inside. Over time, that force can generate a lot more wear to damaged cartilage on the inside of your knee. A reduction in pain causes an increase in the loads at the knee in patients with medial compartment arthritis. When there is a significant increase in inward knee movement, there are substantial effects on the medial compartment of the knee. This detrimental overloading of an arthritic joint, made possible by pain relief, may lead to what is termed an analgesic arthropathy. Dr. Eric Radin believes that anti-inflammatory drugs actually speed the process of deterioration of a joint. He says that when you take pain relievers for arthritis, "you don't have the buzzer going off; the buzzer is called pain."

Researchers are also concerned that pain relievers may impair the ability of the cartilage to repair itself. In animals, hydrocortisone, aspirin, indomethacin, and ibuprofen have all produced significant inhibition of the ability of cartilage to produce the building blocks it needs to repair itself. NSAIDs may also blunt the repair capacity of the key cells in cartilage called chondrocytes.

Studies like these have fired a warning shot across the bow. Many of us who take chronic pain medication for wear and tear may suffer more wear and tear if we kill the pain without changing the underlying process. I know; I used to take twelve or more Advils a day. I absolutely *loved* the stuff—and still do for acute pain. However, I'm concerned enough about the damage I may be doing that I now take none on a regular basis. I'm afraid that pain relievers turn off my body's early-warning system: pain! There is an alternative view. One study shows that certain NSAIDs can interfere with the enzyme responsible for destroying joint cartilage, but it is preliminary and not accepted by most rheumatologists. On a purely practical note, if you take pain relievers for days at a time, as recommended by the FDA, rather than months, you're unlikely to do any long-term damage. So don't hesitate to get proper control of your pain in the short term, but do look for long-term plans that will minimize your risk of drug-induced arthropathy.

The great irony is that there is nothing that a traditional pain reliever can do to slow the progress of wear and tear or osteoarthritis. And as we've just seen, there is the possibility they could make matters worse, although long-term studies are needed to prove the point. But who wants to take the chance?

What if there was a way to have the best of both worlds—kill the pain and *help* your joints? In two randomized controlled trials a supplement called glucosamine was compared to ibuprofen for its ability to relieve pain. Glucosamine was superior in one and equivalent in the other. But glucosamine isn't just a pain reliever. It's also what is termed a "disease-modifying agent." That is, glucosamine may modify the underlying disease process by slowing or even stopping cartilage loss. Not only is there little risk of hurting your joints, there's good evidence you may be making them better. We'll learn more about glucosamine and other disease-modifying agents in the next chapter.

One expert from the Arthritis Foundation has been quoted as

saying that glucosamine and its companion nutritional supplement, chondroitin, are now used by millions of people with osteoarthritis. You may also want to consult the Arthritis Foundation's excellent series of guides. You can find these at www.arthritis.org.

Where does that leave traditional pain relievers? Since disease-modifying supplements may take weeks to work and since the steps recommended in this book may also take weeks to work, using these pain relievers is perfectly reasonable to hold you over. Also, if you have really severe arthritis, you have little choice except joint replacement. My advice is to get your pain under control first. If the traditional pain relievers in this chapter are all that can control your pain, remember that being active far outweighs whatever further risk there is to the joint. Dr. David Felson weighs in that the "benefits of exercise *so* outweigh the harm. You cannot worry about NSAIDs. The best way to be sure there is no harm is to pick joint-friendly sports so you can keep active with little risk." For example, if you take large doses of ibuprofen so you can walk five miles a day on hard concrete with leather-soled shoes, you're probably damaging your joints further. But if you take ibuprofen to relieve pain in your joints so you can participate in a yoga program or bicycle, you're doing a lot more good than harm. My advice is to try to contain your pain first with whatever pain relievers are necessary, then move on to measures that can help you beat wear and tear such as disease-modifying drugs, yoga, and strength training. After you've controlled the pain, try to reduce the dosage. You want to get to the point that you're using NSAIDs on an as-needed basis, rather than taking a fixed dose every day.

7

Protect Your Joints

The locker room of the LA Sports Club at Rockefeller Center is as close to heaven as a locker room can get: elegant wood-paneled lockers, comforting wall-to-wall carpet, the classical strains of Mozart. Enjoying the serenity was a money manager from Rockefeller Plaza who was toweling off after a hard workout. He casually pulled a big bottle of pain relievers from his locker, took a handful of caplets, and threw his head back as he tossed them into his mouth. His eyes caught mine. "Yes?" he queried. "Something the matter?"

"A little pain?" I asked.

"Yes, my knees are killing me."

"Did you know you could be doing yourself more harm than good?"

"You must be joking," he said, clearly upset. He had the haunted, hungry look of someone who lived for the stuff.

"Seriously, the pain may help protect your joints by preventing you from overloading them. In fact, a Rush-Presbyterian-St. Luke's Medical Center study concluded that 'pain may cause patients to alter how they perform activities to decrease the loads on the joints.' "

"Huh? So how could pain relievers be harmful?"

"Simply put, the decrease in pain you enjoy may allow you to load up the part of the joint already damaged by arthritis. The fear is that the pain relief may allow you to further damage your joints."

"Boy, I bet the pharmaceutical companies are just delighted about that."

"Well, I've talked to them and they're quick to point out that no one has actually *proven* that the arthritis does get worse. However, it certainly doesn't get any better. It may be the only major disease in modern medicine for which there are no pharmaceuticals that affect the disease process itself."

His face fell. "So what should I do?"

"Consider disease-modifying agents."

"Huh?"

"Disease-modifying agents can slow, stop, or even reverse the damage in your joints. It's not a very elegant term and hides their true promise. The truth is, there have been *no* prescription medicines to date that slow the destruction of the cartilage in your joints."

The conventional wisdom: Supplements are snake oil.

The real deal: Medical journals don't lie; supplements are finally getting good press.

A ROAD MAP

We'll look at two highly popular disease-modifying agents, glucosamine and chondroitin. We'll also take a look ahead to several promising disease-modifying agents in the pipeline and a novel surgical technique.

THE BEST EVIDENCE THAT SUPPLEMENTS WORK

The traditional medical community often heckles the world of alternative medicine with cries of "Show me the science!" And well they should. In the case of disease-modifying agents, the science is here!

There are fifteen controlled studies showing that supplements may reduce pain, but what's gotten everyone's attention, including the Arthritis Foundation's, is a major study in the British journal *The Lancet* showing that one of them, glucosamine, may actually slow the rate at which cartilage is worn away. Glucosamine sulfate is a component of normal human cartilage. Commercial glucosamine is made from the shells of shrimp, crabs, or lobsters. Sales of glucosamine are estimated to have reached at least $327 million annually in the United States.

The researchers randomly divided 212 patients with arthritis into two groups. One group was given 1,500 milligrams of oral glucosamine sulfate. The other group got a sham treatment. Both groups took their treatments daily for three years. So what happened? Fast-forward to three years later. Doctors carefully compared the knee X rays of those taking glucosamine to participants in the sham-treatment group. The bottom line? Those taking glucosamine sulfate had lost a minuscule 0.06 millimeters from the cartilage in their knee over the three years. That translates to no significant joint space loss detected in those taking glucosamine. Just as important, those taking glucosamine experienced a 20 to 25 percent improvement in pain and disability and an "increased ability to use the affected joint to carry out daily activities," while the sham group had a slight worsening of their symptoms. The people who received the sham treatment lost an average of 0.31 millimeters, five times as much joint space loss.

Boston University Medical Center arthritis expert Tim McAlindon called *The Lancet* article a landmark. "Scarce currency has been given to the notion that progression of osteoarthritis could be retarded pharmacologically, let alone by a nutritional product," he said. "I think it will have a big impact at least in bringing the idea forward to the medical community—and in fact everybody—that we should be looking for interventions which make a difference to osteoarthritis progression. From my perspective it's a very important study on that basis."

When you shop for glucosamine, you'll often find it combined with chondroitin sulfate. For instance, Cosamin DS is a combination of glucosamine hydrochloride and low-molecular-weight chondroitin sulfate. Could adding chondroitin deliver an additional benefit?

While many researchers are impressed by the glucosamine research, they remain unconvinced by the chondroitin research, the most convincing of which is in rabbits. That research showed that addition of chondroitin to glucosamine had a synergistic effect on stimulating the manufacture of a key component of cartilage in the rabbit's knees. The result? In the glucosamine group there were still some areas of moderate and even severe damage. In the group taking glucosamine and chondroitin sulfate there was no severe damage and less moderate damage. While this needs to be confirmed in humans, it is an encouraging sign.

Where does that leave you? Should you consider a therapy that is not completely proven? Here is my own personal opinion. The risk of taking these supplements appears to be very low—far lower than that of traditional pain relievers. So if you take them for pain alone and they work, you've lowered your risk of experiencing an adverse event as a result of taking a traditional pain reliever. The other risk, though, is this: What if they *do* work and work really well? If you don't take them, each year you will lose more cartilage that you won't be able to replace. That's a risk I'm unwilling to take. I want to get in on a good thing early, like a very promising stock. In surveying practitioners, I've found many mainstream rheumatologists, physiatrists, and internists who are recommending that their patients consider these supplements. Some doctors at top institutions such as Johns Hopkins and the Hospital for Special Surgery recommend them as first-choice drugs for mild to moderate wear-and-tear arthritis.

They also have the preliminary backing of the prestigious Arthritis Foundation: "There is emerging evidence to suggest that glucosamine is an appropriate treatment for people with osteo-arthritis (OA) of the knee, providing a number of benefits such as symptom relief, functional improvement and reduction of the progression of cartilage damage."

The Arthritis Foundation urges anyone who is considering the use of glucosamine to consult a physician about how the supplement fits into a comprehensive treatment plan, as do I.

This study hasn't convinced everyone, though. Dr. Stephen E. Straus, director of the National Institutes of Health's National Center for Complementary and Alternative Medicine, underscores the critical public health need to test these agents in a rigorous way: "The National Center for Complementary and Alternative Medicine and NIAMS [National Institute of Arthritis and Musculoskeletal and Skin Diseases] have jointly initiated the largest multicenter study to date of glucosamine and chondroitin sulfate in order to provide Americans with definitive answers about their effectiveness for osteoarthritis." The University of Utah School of Medicine is coordinating a nine-center study of more than one thousand patients. The National Center for Complementary and Alternative Medicine and NIAMS currently have a trial under way that will examine the effects of glucosamine, chondroitin sulfate, and the combination of glucosamine and chondroitin in a crucial $14 million study. This is an important question because glucosamine and chondroitin are often sold together. The results of this study are expected in March 2005.

To add further ammunition to the argument, a Boston University team reviewed thirty-seven studies of the compounds going back more than three decades. Of these, fifteen trials published between 1980 and 1998 met their criteria: double-blind, randomized, placebo-controlled trials that lasted four or more weeks. Only one of the fifteen trials was completely independent of manufacturer support.

I've been very disappointed when friends and family members see their doctors and are dissuaded from trying these supplements. I lost a lot of ground myself by not taking glucosamine in the years before the *Lancet* study was published. One week I'd believe the critics; the next I'd see a promising new study. I took glucosamine or chondroitin on a highly irregular basis. Little wonder the supplements never really took hold! Once the *Lancet* paper appeared, I determined to dig in for real: I began taking the full 1,500 milligrams of glucosamine religiously on a daily basis with 1,200 milligrams of chondroitin. I was amazed at the difference after only a few weeks. My yoga program had taken away all the ache and real pain, but a full-bore glucosamine-and-chondroitin program made my joints feel like silk. The last twinges of hip pain vanished.

Even if you have no pain, I'd encourage you to look at taking supplements as a preventive measure. Here's why. The majority of patients with wear-and-tear arthritis visible on X rays have no pain! Yet each year that goes by, a little more cartilage is worn away. Then one morning you do wake up with pain and without much cartilage left. That's why I recommend early aggressive therapy upon the earliest signs of wear and tear or if you have substantial risk factors such as those conditions we discussed in Chapters 1, 3, and 5. You'll certainly want to see if your physician agrees with me before you start.

What do the pharmaceutical companies think of these supplements? Heresy? I thought they'd be incensed by the very idea of analgesic neuropathy and was anxious about approaching them. I was surprised by quite a reasonable approach. I interviewed Anthony Temple, Ph.D., vice president of medical and regulatory science for the McNeil Consumer & Specialty Pharmaceuticals Division of McNeil-PPC, Inc. He said, "It's appropriate and reasonable to take glucosamine for joint health. On an 'as-needed' basis, you may want to take a conventional pain reliever, but you don't need to keep taking them. *Not* year in, year out." He recommends the idea of parallel treatments: taking either Tylenol and ibuprofen for immediate pain relief and a supplement such as glucosamine for the longer term. He also points out that damage to the key cell in cartilage, the chondrocyte, is probably affected at doses higher than the consumer receives in over-the-counter formulations. In other words, it's the high-dose prescription medications he's most concerned about. Since your first objective is pain relief, don't feel intimidated about taking conventional pain relievers as a first step. Over a month or so, it's unlikely you'll be doing any real damage to your joints. However, try to wean yourself off as the other key measures in this book take hold. You'll find that you do require less and less pain medication.

Glucosamine or other disease-modifying agents don't work right away, so you may have to rely on conventional pain relievers until they kick in.

HOW DO SUPPLEMENTS WORK?

The question is, How on earth do they work when they're just simple building blocks of cartilage? The emerging answer is that they appear to have a much more sophisticated role. Recent studies show they reduce the effect of powerful joint toxins such as nitrous oxide by an incredibly sophisticated effect on cellular messengers called "inflammatory cytokines." Some inflammatory cytokines play a pivotal role in the destruction of cartilage, helping to suppress the manufacture of collagen, a key component of cartilage. The preservation of joint cartilage may be explained by the glucosamine's blocking action on these cellular messengers.

JOINT FUEL

You'll see glucosamine and chondroitin promoted as "joint fuel" to improve performance in athletes. How well they work isn't known scientifically, but there is a new survey showing that athletic trainers get positive results from using glucosamine dietary supplements.

The survey was commissioned by McNeil Consumer Healthcare group in cooperation with the National Athletic Trainers' Association (NATA). Nine of ten athletic trainers received reports of improved joint function from athletes who used glucosamine supplements. One thousand professional athletic trainers were surveyed.

A related survey of professional football athletic trainers reported that players using glucosamine supplements reported benefits in three main areas, including the knees, shoulders, and neck.

The rationale for "joint fuel" working is that glucosamine may play a role in the production of synovial fluid, necessary for joint lubrication.

WHY DO SUPPLEMENTS FAIL TO WORK IN SOME PEOPLE?

I run into a lot of people who say, "Hey! The stuff just plain doesn't work." I've heard it a thousand times. Then I gently probe the user: "How long have you taken it for?" "Oh, a couple of days" is the usual answer. This includes my parents, who both had side effects within a day of trying a cheap drugstore brand of glucosamine. Most users simply fail to commit to a long enough course to feel any effect. They expect them to work like an aspirin or ibuprofen—in hours, not weeks or months. I'd like to see you give them a good six- to eight-week commitment to determine if they work for you. Second, most users limit the amount they take so that they get a suboptimal dose. The daily doses that experts recommend are:

◆ 1,200 mg chondroitin
◆ 1,500 mg glucosamine

This was true for me the first time I took glucosamine. I took a couple of tablets a day but never checked the dose! Once I took the correct amount, I could really feel the effect.

The third reason many fail to get an effect is that they're taking substandard products. Dr. Natalie Eddington of the University of Maryland School of Pharmacy in Baltimore was one of the first to undertake a chemical analysis of popular chondroitin and glucosamine supplements. Here's what really alarmed me: she found that only five of thirty-two Chondroitin brands contained what they claimed! The other twenty-seven had less than 90 percent of what the label claimed, many far less. She claims there is also a lot of variability from one bottle to the next. In another study, many of the chondroitin products failed. Many products had less than 20 percent of what the label claimed! Combination products, that is, products that contained both chondroitin and glucosamine, did badly as well. Forty percent failed in one study. The good news is that glucosamine products are pretty close to the mark.

These products are not cheap. Many Americans have to stretch their budgets to buy them and don't want to find out they're blowing their hard-earned money on junk! The good news is that ConsumerLab.com tests these products so you can be certain you're getting what you paid for. Each product is tested at up to three independent labs. What's more, different batches of the product are tested to be sure the product is consistent from bottle to bottle and from store to store.

Here are some of the products that did pass muster in recent testing. As you can see, they are highly reputable companies—either pharmaceutical companies such as McNeil Consumer Healthcare or high-quality supplement manufacturers such as Schiff. ConsumerLab.com has graciously allowed me to include several products from its list.

Combination Products
- Double Strength Cosamin DS (500 mg glucosamine HCl, 400 mg chondroitin sulfate, 5 mg manganese) (Nutramax)
- Move Free (500 mg glucosamine, 400 mg chondroitin) (Schiff)

Glucosamine-Only Products
- Aflexa (340 mg glucosamine) McNeil Consumer Healthcare
- One-A-Day Joint Health (500 mg glucosamine sulfate) (Bayer)

- Nature Made Glucosamine (500 mg sulfate and HCl) (Natrol)

Chondroitin Sulfate–Only Products

- NOW chondroitin sulfate (600 mg) (Now Foods)

For the complete list, log on to: www.consumerlab.com.

If you don't want to take pills, there are several novel forms, including gum, candy, juice, and energy bars. You'll want to see when they are tested to be sure they pass muster. Some of these products may be pretty high in calories.

SIDE EFFECTS

Indigestion, Nausea

You may possibly have a reaction if you're allergic to shellfish. If you're taking prescription medications, check with your physician about possible cross-sensitivities, especially to diuretics or sulfonamides.

Sulfonamide Sensitivity

To be on the safe side, for patients with sulfonamide sensitivity, it's smart to start with a minimal dose and look for any effects or reactions.

Growth Changes in the Prostate

Some experimental studies show that an increase in chondroitin sulfate levels in prostatic stroma might be associated with hyperplastic or growth changes.

Hypertension

Chondroitin sulfate may contain up to 84 milligrams of sodium. This amount represents only 2 to 8 percent of the standard amount of sodium intake when you're restricted. Still, you need to be aware of the extra sodium intake.

Mad Cow Disease (Bovine Spongiform Encephalopathy)

Chondroitin comes from cattle trachea (windpipes). You'll hear speculation through the grapevine about the connection between mad cow disease and chondroitin. Dr. Tim McAlindon states, "The major supplement makers say they are not using cattle tissue from countries with BSE, but experts point out there's no system in place to monitor what actually goes into supplements, leaving room for error." There is much less supervision and regulation of nutritional products than there is of pharmaceutical products. Dr. McAlindon continues that "manufacturers import raw ingredients from overseas from places like China and encapsulate them. So you never know when buying a product off the shelf where the original material came from or how well the cattle from which it came were treated. It is a bit concerning, I think."

Although the infectious agent that causes bovine spongiform encephalopathy (BSE) is not normally found in cartilage, critics speculate that it might possibly contaminate cartilage in the slaughterhouse. However, as long as the material is manufactured and handled correctly, these products should be safe from mad cow disease.

Bleeding

Claudia L. Thomas, M.D., of the Johns Hopkins University Department of Orthopaedics, writes, "Over-the-counter 'arthritis' medications like Cosamin generally contain glucosamine and chondroitin sulfate. Many patients report significant relief of arthritis pain as a result of taking these medications, above and beyond the beneficial effects of placebo.

"It is a commonly held opinion that Cosamin and other glucosamine and chondroitin sulfate compounds do not have any associated bleeding risks, but recent investigations abroad have suggested that they do. These over-the-counter medications seem to have some adverse effect on the blood's ability to clot, due to interference with a clotting function called platelet aggregation. Similar effects on platelets have been observed with other anti-inflammatory medications. This means that patients taking a glucosamine/chondroitin sulfate compound may be at increased risk of gastrointestinal and other bleeding, similar to the increased bleeding risks that have been associated with other anti-inflammatory medications. For this reason, many surgeons recommend that these compounds be discontinued prior to elective surgery, to reduce the risk of excessive bleeding."

Despite these precautions, Dr. McAlindon concludes, "I should say these compounds seem incredibly safe compared to NSAIDs."

WARNINGS

Four groups of patients should be cautious when considering these products.

Diabetics

There is a concern that glucosamine may increase your blood sugar level. If you have diabetes, monitor your blood sugar level carefully for the first month you take glucosamine to determine if your blood sugar levels are higher than normal. Also, there is concern that glucosamine may cause insulin resistance. In fact, glucosamine was used a few decades ago in an experiment to cause insulin-resistance diabetes in rats. The rats were given a very high dose intravenously. It worked! Their insulin resistance increased. However, it appears very unlikely that the much smaller oral doses used for arthritis would have that effect. If you do have diabetes, to be cautious, be sure to check your blood sugar levels to make certain the control of your diabetes is not worsened. Dr. McAlindon suggests, "If someone has a family history of diabetes but themselves is not diabetic, then they should be a bit careful." Diabetics should always check with a doctor before considering these products!

Regular Users of Anticoagulants

Regular users of anticoagulants or daily aspirin therapy should have their blood-clotting times checked when taking chondroitin since it could alter blood-clotting activity. Its molecular structure is said to be similar to that of heparin, a potent blood thinner.

People with Liver Disease

These people may want to minimize additional manganese intake from supplements. One brand had higher-than-normal amounts of manganese. For that reason, check the ConsumerLab.com site for products that do not contain high levels of manganese.

People Who Are Allergic to Shellfish

Glucosamine is extracted from shellfish, making it potentially unsafe for those with shellfish allergies. If you are allergic to shellfish, consult your doctor before deciding to take glucosamine. However, in many cases, allergies are caused by the proteins in the shellfish and not the carbohydrate chitin, from which the glucosamine comes.

WHICH PRODUCT SHOULD YOU TAKE?

Purists take glucosamine, which has the best available evidence to date. Optimists may want to take glucosamine and chondroitin since the hope is that the two work synergistically.

OTHER DISEASE-MODIFYING AGENTS

Diacerein

Here's a medication that goes right to the heart of the problem. Interleukin-1 (IL-1) is the gang leader in your body's attack on its own joints. IL-1 orchestrates and directs a variety of agents that can eat away at your cartilage.

Diacerein inhibits the synthesis of interleukin-1. Its effectiveness has been proven in animal studies, but then you and I aren't lab rats. Even though you've probably heard very little about diacerein, there are real and impressive results in human beings. To be specific, a total of 482 patients were evaluated; 269 patients were given diacerein, the rest a placebo. X rays were used to evaluate the degree of joint narrowing that occurred over the course of a year. Among the 269 patients, the annual joint-space-narrowing rate was significantly lower in those receiving diacerein than in those receiving no drugs. Those taking diacerein lost 0.18 millimeters per year, while those taking the placebo lost 0.23 millimeters per year. Diacerein is also a decent pain reliever, as shown by an earlier Canadian study. It is not FDA-approved but is approved in some European countries. Some American doctors are writing prescriptions for American patients who then have their prescriptions filled in Europe and air-shipped to the United States.

Early human trials show that pain relief is similar to that of NSAIDs but takes longer to take effect. The optimal daily dosage of diacerein for patients with knee osteoarthritis is 100 milligrams per day (50 milligrams twice daily). Mild to moderate diarrhea is the most frequent side effect, increasing with the dosage.

Dr. Marc Hochberg summarizes the latest findings: "Diacerein is a slow-acting symptomatic arthritis drug which in studies conducted in Europe has been shown to be effective in patients with hip and knee osteoarthritis. In addition, the Echodiah study [an evaluation of the chondromodulating effect of diacerein in osteoarthritis of the hip] demonstrated that it had structure-modifying activity in patients with hip osteoarthritis. My understanding is that the French health agency has allowed the company to include this on the label. In addition, the results of the study have been published in high-quality peer review journals. At this time, my comment would be that the results need to be confirmed in a second study and that additional studies need to be conducted to see if has structure-modifying results in knee osteoarthritis. It is not available in the U.S., but there is a phase 3 trial only for symptom effects in knee osteoarthritis being conducted in North America."

Ademetionine (SAM-e)

Another disease-modifying drug, ademetionine, also known as SAM-e (discussed on page 86), is a particular form of the amino acid metionine known as S-adenosylmethionine. This amino acid is manufactured in the body and can be found in many tissues. Rather than X rays, researchers chose a novel and high-tech way of evaluating its effectiveness. Researchers at the Free University of Berlin looked at the signal intensity from the joint on an MRI. They found a "highly significant correlation" between an increase in cartilage signal intensity and clinical improvement. This did not, however, extend to all patients in the treatment group.

Tetracycline

There are two major building blocks of cartilage, aggrecan and collagen, which give cartilage its stiffness and strength.

In wear-and-tear arthritis, the turnover rates of these building blocks increase as they are broken down and discarded. That has led scientists to look for a way of inhibiting this breakdown. To do so they have targeted the enzymes that cause the breakdown in the hope that they can slow or even arrest the progression of arthritis. One drug that does this is doxycycline. Although designed as an antibiotic, doxycycline is also a potent inhibitor of several enzymes that break down cartilage. In animals with osteoarthritis, the drug reduces joint damage. For that reason, a trial of the drug in humans is now under way. Experts hope that the clinical trial confirms that doxycycline may prevent the development of wear-and-tear arthritis in unaffected joints and prevent the progression of the disease in joints already affected.

Dr. Ken Brandt, professor of medicine and head of Rheumatology at Indiana University and director of the Indiana University Multipurpose Arthritis and Musculoskeletal Diseases Center, is the lead investigator of this study. The study is under way and patients have been treated, but Dr. Brandt doesn't expect to have any progress or results to report for another year.

Arthritis expert Tim McAlindon is hopeful that doxycycline will prove to be an effective disease-modifying drug because there is some good basic science reasoning that it might be.

Hormone Replacement Therapy

HRT may prevent women from developing wear-and-tear arthritis in their knees. Researchers in Australia say that the estrogen in HRT tablets may help to stop the loss of cartilage. However, this is not reason enough to begin HRT. In consultation with your physician, you'll want to look at the full spectrum of potential benefits and newfound risks.

Repair Cartilage

Swedish researchers have reported a novel cell transplant technique. Here's how it works. First, the investigators removed cartilage cells from a healthy part of an injured knee that had suffered the loss of a small piece of cartilage. Second, they grew the cells in the laboratory for about three weeks. Third, they then injected them into the defective portion of the cartilage, usually a small divot, and covered it with a small piece of periosteum, the tissue that normally covers bone. The result? Clinically, the pain, swelling, and knee locking were reduced. Two years later, the regenerated cartilage looked much like normal tissue. Fourteen of the sixteen patients had good to excellent results. Ongoing studies are looking at how to best identify who will benefit. More than four thousand patients have benefited to date. Most health care plans will pay for the procedure for appropriate patients. Remember, once badly damaged, joint cartilage does not normally regenerate. In addition to causing pain and restricted mobility, chronic injuries to joint cartilage may lead to further deterioration of the joint surface. For further information, call Genzyme Biosurgery at (800) 453-6948 or visit www.carticel.com.

ARTHRITIS FOUNDATION RECOMMENDATIONS

The Arthritis Foundation urges anyone who is considering the use of disease-modifying agents to consult a physician about how they fit within a comprehensive treatment plan. I don't rely on disease-modifying agents alone and don't recommend that you do either.

Yoga, strength training, and the right footwear all had a big effect on my disease. A comprehensive treatment package gives you your best assurance that you're going to get significantly better. In considering the use of disease-modifying drugs, the Arthritis Foundation makes the following important recommendations.

Stay on your other medications. Supplements should be taken along with your current medication and not be considered as replacements for known and effective therapies. If your current treatment plan isn't working or is causing side effects, ask your doctor to suggest other options. Quitting some medications abruptly can cause problems; quitting others can cause your condition or symptoms to worsen.

Do the research. Learn as much as you can about the supplement you are considering. Find evidence that the supplement is effective in arthritis. Learn about its known side effects and potential interaction with other supplements or medications. Seek reliable sources of information, such as your doctor, pharmacist, scientific studies, and so on.

Consult your doctor. There are more than a hundred types of arthritis. Some supplements, such as glucosamine, are helpful for specific types of arthritis. Find out what type of arthritis you have and talk to your doctor about supplements you are considering. Ask his advice and if he will help you monitor the effects.

Ask your doctor about dosage. If you decide to take glucosamine or other supplements, follow the directions specified by the manufacturer or consult your doctor about the proper dosage.

Avoid combining supplements. Avoid taking multiple supplements because you can't be certain which supplement may be helping and which hurting.

Stick with a reputable manufacturer. Choose products sold by large, well-established companies. If you don't recognize a brand name, ask about the company's reputation, how long it has been in the business, and how long the store has stocked the brand.

Report side effects to your doctor. Report adverse side effects quickly to your doctor and stop taking the product. In addition, alert the FDA at (800) 332-1088 or www.fda.gov/medwatch and notify the manufacturer. The FDA relies on consumer and physician reports to catch problems.

You can find more information from the Arthritis Foundation on its Web site, www.arthritis.org.

Disease-modifying drugs are a revolution in the treatment of wear and tear. For the first time in medical history, there is the hope that the damage to joint cartilage can be slowed, stopped, or even reversed. The addition of disease-modifying drugs to your program of recovery is a cornerstone upon which to build new strength, flexibility, and power to turn back the clock on the degeneration that makes so many of us look and feel old.

8

Fix the Flaws

What could possibly be a better buffer against wear and tear than the high technology coming out of Beaverton, Oregon; Penn State; or even MIT? What could be an easier way to beat wear and tear than just buying a pair of shoes? They're a cheap, easy way to decrease the wear and tear inflicted by excess body weight, muscle weakness, heavy heel pounding, and many fatal flaws.

I started my own personal quest at a traditional shoe store, where there was an entire section of dress shoes with Nike running shoe technology embedded in them. You might call them stealth shoes. I tried both a loafer and a more formal shoe. The loafer had a little harsher heel strike but seemed to contain my foot roll better.

However, I opted for the dress shoe model so I could feel the full effect of the cushioning. I laced them up and walked out of the store to have dinner with my wife. The heel was squishy, like walking on an air ball. But then I noticed something odd: it seemed to force my whole body forward, pushing me off my heel so that I had to use more of my quadriceps as my foot landed on the ground during a normal stride.

Pretty soon, I was pleased. I could walk faster, with some spring put back into my step. The shoes fixed another problem, foot slap. With a leather-soled, hard-heeled shoe, after heel strike the entire shoe tends to slap down on the ground. Foot slap can lead to shin-splints, among other conditions. The Nikes eliminated this and allowed for a slower, more controlled rollout. I met my wife for dinner at Orsay, an elegant Parisian restaurant on Seventy-third Street and Lexington Avenue. We sat side by side. In my excitement, I lifted my shoe up just above the table and showed it to my wife. "Oh, Bob," she said, "don't ever wear those with any of our friends. They'll think you have a handicap." The next day she saw my new shoes on the floor at home. She grabbed them, threw them in the trash chute, and said again, "You're *not* wearing those around *my* friends!" I recovered them from the building superintendent. Now I wear them everywhere: running, hiking, and—yes—to dinner with friends!

The conventional wisdom: These shoes are really cute.
The real deal: They're killing your joints.

If there's one take-home point to be gained from this chapter, it's this: wear a high-tech running or walking shoe for everyday activities that accommodates the problems we saw in Chapter 3. After reading that chapter you should have a pretty good idea of what you need. In this chapter you'll learn what shoes can do for you and find solutions to problems you may have uncovered earlier in this book.

Which shoes should you try? Despite all the science, the final selection is still made based on educated trial and error. Peter Cavanaugh is the most famous shoe researcher in the world and a friend of mine from my days in sports medicine. Peter is a professor at Penn State and has run a large shoe lab there for years. He said that for an individual runner, there is no scientific way of determining what shoe to get; you just have to try them out. However, he says this does not deny that such a selection could be made in the lab. And that's exactly what I did. Make a list of shoes that look promising for you. Go to the biggest and best running shoe or walking store you can. Try on three or four different models of different brands. Go on the treadmill at the store or ask if you can take your final selections to a gym where you can try them on the treadmill without scuffing the sole. Then make your determination based on how good they make you feel! *Runner's World* thoroughly reviews different shoe criteria. These are what you'll be looking at in a good running shoe store. You'll also find the recommendations of the American Academy of Podiatric Sports Medicine (AAPSM). The AAPSM comes out annually with a list of athletic shoe recommendations that are recognized by the prestigious American College of Sports Medicine. The AAPSM criteria can be seen at www.aapsm.org/crishoe.html.

The lists of running shoes may seem daunting, even overwhelming. There are, however, just three basic shoe types. Let's take a brief look at them and then address the specific problems from Chapter 3, "Fatal Flaws."

MOTION CONTROL SHOES

If you tested as a high roller in Chapter 3, this may be the first shoe you want to try.

They are recommended for runners who are moderate to severe overpronators. These shoes typically give you maximum control of your rear foot and provide the extra support on the arch side of your shoe to stop your foot from rolling. Examples are the New Balance 854, the Asics 2070, and the Nike Air Structure Triax, which are shoes that deliver moderate stability without a heavy, clunky feel. Duplicating the success of these styles are the Asics Gel-MC Plus V, Nike's Air Equilibrium, and the redesigned Brooks Beast.

The AAPSM further divides motion control shoes into three categories:

Running Shoes: Mild Motion Control
- ◆ Adidas Cairo (M/W)
- ◆ Adidas Brevard (M/W)
- ◆ Asics 2070 (M/W)
- ◆ Asics Gel-Kayano VII (M/W)

- Brooks Adrenaline (M/W)
- Brooks Vapor (M/W)
- Brooks Trance (M/W)
- New Balance 854 (M/W)
- New Balance 763 (M/W)
- New Balance 999 (M/W)
- New Balance 1220 (M/W)
- Nike Air Structure Triax (M/W)
- Nike Durham and Nike Kantara (M/W)

Running Shoes: Moderate Motion Control

- Adidas Piedmont (M/W)
- Asics Gel-Foundation III (M/W)
- Asics Nandi trail shoe (M/W)
- Brooks Addiction IV (M/W)
- Brooks Gila trail shoe (M/W)
- New Balance 587 (M/W)
- Reebok Supreme Control DMX (M/W)
- Saucony GRID Hammer (M/W)

Running Shoes: Maximum Motion Control

- Asics Gel-MC Plus V (M/W)
- Brooks Beast (M/W)
- Brooks Ariel (W) (Note: somewhat less control than Beast)
- New Balance 1121 (M/W)
- Saucony GRID Stabil Classic (M/W)
- Reebok Ventilator DMX (M/W)

CUSHIONED SHOES

If you tested as having a high-arched cavus foot in Chapter 3, this is the first shoe for you to try. They are recommended by the AAPSM for runners who need maximum cushioning and minimum medial arch support. They're also a great solution if you are a heavy heel striker or have excess body weight.

Running Shoes: Cushioned

◆ Asics Gel-Cumulus III
◆ Asics Gel-Nimbus II
◆ Mizuno Wave Rider

STABILITY SHOES

I quickly felt that cushioning was a godsend; that is, until I found that my foot was rolling all over the place, creating more problems than it solved. There is a trade-off between cushioning and motion control. As Kenneth Holt of Boston University states, "You want to have shock absorption, but at the same time you need to have control. If you have someone who has a structural problem, then limiting the amount of pronation and the lateness of the pronation that occurs is more critical than good shock absorption. The recommendation is to go with a motion control shoe and not a shock-absorbing shoe." The ideal compromise is a stability shoe, which has medial arch side support to prevent excessive roll and still has good midsole cushioning. Dr. Peter Cavanaugh confirmed what I was finding: "The two general things that are talked about in athletic footwear are the issue of cushioning and the issue of control. And many people feel that those two issues are likely to be competing and that you either have one or you have the other." Not true! Get a stability shoe.

Stability shoes are best suited to runners who are mild to moderate overpronators and/or who need added support and durability.

OTHER IMPORTANT SHOE FEATURES

Here are some other key features you should look for:

Dual-Density Soles

A dual-density sole has softer material on the outside and firmer material on the inside. Why? When your foot lands on the ground during a normal stride, you come down on the soft side, allowing for shock absorption. As your foot rolls inward, it rolls onto the harder material, which limits pronation.

In addition, if the structural problem is in the forefoot, the harder material has to go all the way up into the forefoot. There are only about two or three shoe manufacturers that actually make a shoe with a full-length dual-density midsole. If you're not a runner, consider this: a tennis or volleyball shoe usually has a more rigid midsole; a higher-density midsole is generally better. "The dual density kind of serves both purposes on the outside when you hit. It absorbs shock, but then, as you roll in, it prevents the excessive motion from occurring," concludes Kenneth Holt.

Heel Counters

The heel counter is the rear part of the shoe, located at the back of the heel above the sole. Its rigid material provides support. To many people this is one of the most important areas of a running shoe. The heel counter is what's going to give you that stability and prevent distortion. Most of the running shoes over the last ten years have added medial/lateral counter supports. This reinforcement is usually plastic and it's built into leather areas on the counter to prevent breakdown.

Socks

Good athletic socks can help absorb moisture and add an element of stability to the foot.

Lacing

If you have a high instep, with a lacing system that goes directly over the bone, you could develop irritation. The worst-case scenario, according to Dr. Jeffrey Ross, lecturing at the American College of Sports Medicine, is that the "nerve can get pinched or irritated and can develop a neuropathy or a neuproxia of that nerve just from the laces."

Be careful in the forefoot as well: "If the laces are too tight, you get a squeeze of the forefoot and what happens? You start to get numbness, or if you have a neuroma, then that neuroma can become symptomatic." A neuroma occurs when two bones in the toes continually rub together. This causes a nerve in your foot to swell, creating a neuroma, or a "pinched nerve." It occurs most commonly between the metatarsal heads of the third and fourth toes.

Size

Here's a guide to proper size. Doctors Pat Nunan and Jeff Ross, mediators of a symposium at the American College of Sports Medicine's annual meeting, recommended a very specific technique: With the person seated, place his or her foot on a piece of paper in front of you and trace around the foot. Measure the tracing to determine the foot's length and width. Measure the distance between the two furthest points of the tracing; this will determine the full length of the foot. Reduce this number by one-fifth of an inch. For width, measure the distance between the two widest points on your tracing, which will usually be the first metatarsal to the fifth metatarsal. Again, reduce this number by one-fifth of an inch.

Now let's take an in-depth look at specific problems and how shoes, braces, wedges, and other devices can help you beat fatal flaws.

PROBLEMS AND SOLUTIONS

PROBLEM: I walk with high impact; I'm a "digger"; I have a cavus foot.

SOLUTION: Cushioned shoes

Fortunately, it doesn't take much to vastly improve how you feel with a good cushioned shoe. Dr. Mario Lafortune, director of the Nike Sports Research Lab, one of the top labs in the industry, says, "It doesn't take much to cushion the load. Nearly any kind of cushion will cut the sharp impact at foot-ground contact." Researchers see an "incredible reduction" of the spike with a running shoe. The rate of loading of the knee falls, too.

PROBLEM: I have a destructive foot; I'm an overpronator.

The "destructive foot" overpronates. That means that as your foot lands on the ground during a normal stride, your midfoot rolls across to the inside. In other words, your arch collapses upon weight bearing. These twisting and torquing forces can drive straight through to the knee and even the hip. Over time, these forces can be very destructive. Look closely at an overpronator, and you'll see that what happens to the forefoot as the heel comes off the ground is that the arch continues to flatten.

SOLUTION: Shoes with dual-density soles

Look for a shoe that has full-length dual-density soles. The Adidas Chiro is one such shoe. Beware of shoes that have just a rear-foot dual density. You want to look for a good shock-absorbing shoe in the heel but a shoe that also prevents excessive pronation in the midfoot, suggests Dr. Cheryl Riegger-Krugh.

SOLUTION: Orthotics

Professor Kenneth Holt says, "You are filling in the space that's between the ground and the foot."

The wedge goes on the inner side to prevent the foot from rolling in either excessively or too late. You can buy over-the-counter orthotics. The following over-the-counter orthotics are recommended by the AAPSM:

- Pro Lab Gold
- Superfeet
- Quickstride

PROBLEM: I have inside knee pain.

Wear and tear to the inside of the knee is nearly ten times as common as isolated pain in the lateral compartment. Here's why. First, during normal gait, many of us have a high load on the medial compartment. Second, there is a fairly high trauma rate to the medial meniscus among individuals who suffered from old football, soccer, basketball, skiing, and other injuries. Third, if you're bowlegged, you direct more of the forces into the inside of your knee. In addition, with each ensuing year you may get more and more bowlegged as cartilage wears away and your lateral ligaments loosen and allow more lateral motion—so you transfer more and more load to your medial knee compartment. Over the years you can wear down this cartilage and suffer from early arthritis. You may be able to delay that by five to ten years with what we know today about prevention.

SOLUTION: Braces

Sure, you've heard of them and seen them, but did you know they can shift the load within your knee to prevent wear and tear? They're made of newer, lighter materials and are ideal if you're young and active with knee pain or in the early stages of arthritis.

Although much of the research has focused on the relief of the medial compartment in bowlegged patients, the brace is also used with lateral compartment and bilateral arthritis. However, the fact is that it actually works better on the lateral side. The lateral and medial knee biomechanics are different. It's much easier to unload the lateral compartment in those who have knock knees than the medial compartment in those who have bowlegs, even though bowlegs are more common.

PROBLEM: I am bowlegged or knock-kneed and have severe problems because of it.

SOLUTION: Tibial osteotomy

This surgical procedure realigns the knee and can be quite successful. The idea is to take a wedge out of the leg to make it straighter and to take the pressure off the knee. Dr. Frank A. Cordasco, orthopedic surgeon at the Hospital for Special Surgery, explains, "Osteotomy straightens the knees of patients who have a significant 'knock-kneed' or 'bowlegged' deformity by removing a small wedge of bone. This corrects the malalignment and allows the relatively normal compartment to receive the increased pressure while taking away stress from the arthritic compartment."

PROBLEM: I have excess pressure on the inside of the knee.
SOLUTION: Wedges

These are a neat low-tech way to take the pressure off the inside of your knee. A wedge fitted on the outside of your shoe, called a lateral shoe wedge, decreases the pressure on your medial knee compartment.

PROBLEM: I love my shoes but still need to correct for a fatal foot flaw.
SOLUTION: Insoles

Here is a simple, cheap, and often effective way to help correct some biomechanical problems by stabilizing the foot: remove the insole that came in your walking or running shoes and replace it with over-the-counter insoles. They can be used to cushion or to support your foot. I get insoles heat-shaped to my foot at my local ski boot store, Inner Boot Works in Stowe, Vermont. They provide excellent support for my high-arched foot and make running, walking, hiking, tennis, and biking easier. They're light and flexible and feel as if they're part of the shoe.

PROBLEM: I don't run but love the running shoe technology and design.
SOLUTION: High-tech walking shoes

The difference between walking shoes and a full-out running shoe is the magnitude of the force you are going to see, says Dr. Lafortune. For instance, Nike uses different pressure and dimensions in the air bag designed for walking shoes. Softer midsoles are generally used in walking shoes. "This gives the user greater comfort because a softer air bag makes it much more comfortable for walking." The lowering of the foot during walking differs in timing from that during running. Also, the force on the bottom of the foot is only half as large during walking as during running. Dr. Lafortune employed a pressure-measuring insole, which recorded a far different pattern in walking than running. For instance, since the forces of walking after the heel strike are lower, you want a more compliant midsole in a walking shoe. In the forefoot the order of loading is different with walking. There is a lower load on the forefoot, and it is spread better across the entire ball of your foot. No sooner did I get off the phone than I decided to act! I'd go out and buy a new pair of walking shoes.

I could barely contain my excitement as I headed off to the Cole Haan store and bought my first pair of walking shoes, the ones I wore to dinner with my wife. The first thing I noticed was that the heel was a lot softer than a running shoe's, almost squishy. The shock absorption is a little clumsy, but I still like them. They have the running shoe air pocket but not the running shoe construction. Once you compress the heel, the shoe can roll straight, left, or right, so you have to apply some direction or learn to land slightly further forward. They worked like a charm. Why was the pain gone so quickly? I'm convinced that less heel pounding made an immediate difference. Podiatrist Dr. Howard Dananberg has an even more interesting take. He uses the term "neurogenic hypersensitivity": if you repeat a painful pattern of walking over and over, it becomes acutely hypersensitive. By altering the way you walk ever so slightly, you notice an immediate drop in pain. I found that change almost immediately just by changing shoes. Even though much of this section is on running shoes, if you don't run, look for high-tech walking shoes that have characteristics better designed for walking. You won't find the same extensive technical reviews for them as for running shoes; nonetheless, there are some great shoes out there. In the "expert picks" below, Patrick Nunan recommends several.

EXPERT PICKS

Shoe selection is very personal. However, I did canvas the best people in the industry to see what they like. Let's take a look.

Mario Lafortune, Director of the Nike Sports Research Laboratory

Picks

◆ **Air Max Healthwalker (walking):** Includes large low-pressure airsoles in both heel and forefoot areas to deliver maximal impact protection to the walker. The forefoot airsole is incorporated in the inboard midsole to enhance the comfort provided by air.

◆ **Air Pure Simplicity (walking):** Sports a new design with a dynamic stretch mesh for a socklike fit. The heel airsole combines with the Phylite midsole to provide lightweight flexibility and great cushioning. With 100 percent of the shoe used, solid rubber pods are strategically located to ensure traction and durability.

◆ **Air Skylon (running):** Midsole and outsole are combined in one piece for lighter weight, more flexibility, and better ride. It has a full-length airsole for cushioning.

◆ **Air Kantara (running):** Has a thick airsole unit for exceptional impact protection in the heel area combined with a forefoot airsole to protect the metatarsal area. The shoe midsole combines a firmer medial phylon and footbridge to control rearfoot movement, pronation. Ideal shoe for the heavier runners.

◆ **Air Structure Triax (running):** Provides an excellent combination of cushioning and motion control in a training shoe. Airsoles in both heel and forefoot areas provide the cushioning. Footbridge added to full-length dual-density midsole for greater stability.

Cheryl Riegger-Krugh, Sc.D., Assistant Professor at the University of Colorado Health Sciences Center

"In general, I recommend that people wear good shock-absorbing running shoes no matter whether they are going to run or not. I have found Nike Air Structure and Brooks Women's Beasts to be good shock-absorbing shoes.

"For people who are repetitive impulse loaders and midfoot pronators, you want a good shock-absorbing shoe in the heel but a shoe that prevents excessive pronation in the midfoot. For people who are repetitive impulse loaders and supinators, you want a good shock-absorbing shoe and one that supports the foot align-ment."

Picks

◆ Nike Air Structure Walk

◆ Brooks Women's Beast

◆ New Balance shoes, because they come in more graded widths, so sometimes people can fit into them better

Kenneth Holt, Associate Professor of Physical Therapy at Boston University's Sargent College of Health and Rehabilitation Sciences

Holt likes full-length dual-density shoes for people with the most common structural abnormality (combined forefoot and rearfoot varus) and sees them as "the best solution if you have a mild pronation problem."

Pick

◆ Adidas Cairo

Consumers Union, the Nonprofit Publisher of Consumer Reports

In the October 1999 issue of *Consumer Reports,* Consumers Union found no clear leader in terms of cushioning in walking shoes. In fact, they found that "after just 20 miles of simulated walking with our mechanical foot, the foam in most shoes' mid-soles stiffened—generally by about 30 percent."

Patrick Nunan, D.P.M., Podiatrist and President of the American Academy of Podiatric Sports Medicine

Picks

◆ **Rockports and Dressports:** Dr. Nunan likes these because they tend to be more stylish, even though they can accommodate orthotics. "The dress shoe by Rockport is probably the best they have out now made in the U.S.," says Nunan. The women's version of the Rockport dress shoe is called the Dressport.

◆ **Asics All Walks:** These are good for casual or dress. They are orthotic-friendly and have a deep, wide toe box. They have a

Gore-Tex outer, so they're great in wet weather. They also have a tread that's almost like a trail shoe but are stylish enough to wear in the office.

◆ **New Balance:** These are great because they have various widths and accommodate orthotics. New Balance makes a pair of slip-ons that actually stay on your foot!

◆ **Naot:** These shoes come with the option of a moldable insole. In addition, the Naot has a deep and wide toe box and also accommodates orthotics. This is a decent-looking women's shoe. The biggest selling point is a thick insole, even in the sandals, which is, again, removable. You can get an impression taken of your foot and have a custom-molded insole put in your shoe, like a semi-orthotic, for a more comfortable, even perfect fit. Some canting can be done. If you wear sandals in the summer and want a better fit, try Naots.

◆ **SAS (San Antonio Shoes):** These shoes are handmade in the United States, and the company makes many different styles especially for women. SAS accommodate orthotics and they are handmade with excellent quality control.

◆ **Mephisto and Ecco:** These are great because they have a wide, deep toe box. The outersole lasts a long time and is made of a high grade of carbon rubber. Women may want to consider Mephisto or Ecco.

OTHER SHOES

Here are the AAPSM's recommendations for cross-training, walking, and aerobic shoes (ranked +1 to +3 according to the amount of motion control).

Cross Training
◆ Asics New Porter (M/W) +2
◆ Asics Mercury (M/W) Volleyball/Cross-trainer +2
◆ Nike Air Bokul Max (M) +3
◆ Nike Air Sokul (M) +2

- ◆ Nike Max Ordeal (W) +2
- ◆ New Balance 1003 (M/W) +2
- ◆ New Balance 661 (M/W) +1/+2
- ◆ New Balance 790 (M/W) Tennis +3
- ◆ New Balance 800 (M/W) +3
- ◆ Adidas Response TRC (M) +2

Walking

- ◆ Brooks WT Leather Addiction (M/W) +3
- ◆ Rockport World Tour (M/W) +2
- ◆ Rockport Prowalker DMX (M/W) +2
- ◆ New Balance 840 Series (M/W) +3
- ◆ New Balance 810 Series (M/W) +2
- ◆ Asics Tech Walker (M/W) +2

Aerobics

- ◆ Nike Tuned Appeal (W)
- ◆ Nike Catena (W)
- ◆ Nike Shatter Mid (W)

Electric Shoes

Want high tech? This is it, the ThinkShoe from VectraSense Technologies. Designer Ronald S. Demon was quoted as saying, "The shoe can basically look at how you move, the pressure distribution on the foot, and adjust how the shoe feels." There is a small computer with seven sensors that continuously sense the pressure being applied by the foot to the shoe. If your foot strike changes, the computer can increase the pressure inside an air bladder. The price? $150.

Dress Shoes

Okay, so you can't be seen at work in a pair of running shoes. What do you do? Forget the traditional dress shoe for all but social occasions and around the office. These create two problems, high impulse loading and foot slap. Foot slap occurs once the heel hits and the rest of the foot follows through. "We see very, very high spikes on the force plate," says Nike lab director Mario Lafortune. Fortunately, there is an attempt by manufacturers to build shoes your family won't throw into the trash bin. Here are a few to try for everyday wear. They won't have all the features of a well-designed running shoe but you can at least get decent shock absorption. They can't do much varus or valgus canting because of the limitations of a dress shoe. For instance, Bally now has a neat-looking black leather shoe, which looks like a highly polished, formal running shoe. They join half a dozen shoe manufacturers. The Cole Haan Nike, in my own experience, had the best shock absorption.

WHAT TO AVOID

Flared Heels

A wide, flared heel can act as a lever to roll your foot quickly and excessively. Let's say you land on the outside of your foot. With a flared heel, your foot will roll more quickly from outside to the inside. Flared heels were once the rage on running shoes, but many runners found that the wide flare around the heel compromised the control of their foot. Try a really squishy wide, flared heel, and you'll find that as you land the shoe can roll pretty much in any direction!

High Heels

High-heeled shoes worn for long periods of time can lead to knee pain. Leading researchers at Harvard Medical School reported in the British journal *The Lancet* that high-heeled shoes may increase the forces on the knee that "may contribute to the development of osteoarthritis." High heels increased the forces on the knee an average of 23 percent, compared to walking barefoot. Those forces were right where they'd do the most damage, on the inner area of the knee, where arthritis more commonly develops in women. Measurements demonstrated increased forces both across the kneecap and the medial compartment of the knee. Not lost on the researchers is the fact that women are twice as prone to wear-and-tear arthritis of the knee as men.

The most potentially harmful kind of high-heeled shoe has a wide heel, sometimes called a chunky heel. The lure of wider-heeled shoes is that they are more comfortable; however, that comfort lures women to wear them all day long, increasing the damage they may do.

Wide-heeled dress shoes are producing even greater amounts of knee-joint torque than narrow-base-high-heeled shoes, creating pressure on the medial knee compartment and the kneecap. Dr. Casey Kerrigan of Harvard Medical School's Department of Physical Medicine and Rehabilitation was quoted by the Associated Press as saying, "I liken it to smoking—one cigarette is not painful, but over a lifetime it is. Wide-heeled shoes feel comfortable, so women wear them all day long. They are better for your feet than stiletto heels, but just as bad for your knees." The authors conclude that wide-heeled high-heeled shoes "do cause abnormal knee torques that are believed to be relevant to the development of knee osteoarthritis." Dr. Kerrigan makes a simple recommendation: "Wear no heels at all. It takes a long time to feel the effects of knee osteoarthritis—and once you do, it's too late." Compared to walking barefoot, chunky high heels increased the pressure on the inside of the knee by 26 percent.

Defective Shoes

Be careful that your shoes don't make your condition worse. Dr. Patrick Nunan warns, "I think there's a big quality control issue with shoes." For example, you may buy a shoe that is already tilting well to the inside. This will cause you to pronate excessively causing more problems rather than solving them.

One way to avoid buying defective shoes is to set the shoes on the table after you take them out of the box. They should be stable and not rock. Also, be sure the heel counter is perpendicular to the midsole and doesn't wobble. Inspect the air bags to be sure they are fully inflated and not leaking. Also, avoid a narrow or very low toe box.

The Wrong Shoes

Shoes control your feet while running. The foot has a natural pattern that it needs to maintain during foot strike and the toe-off or propulsive stage. The wrong shoe for you can change this pattern and alter the stress from the feet all the way up to the hips and lower back. One clue that you're wearing the wrong shoes is pain in the ankles, shins, knees, or hips. Also look for blisters, bruised toenails, a heel that slips as you walk, pain along the bottom of your foot, or the development of neuromas. Be wary of shock-absorbing shoes that sacrifice stability or control, warns professor of physical therapy Kenneth Holt: "Soft shoes exacerbate the potential to overpronate and change the timing of pronation. . . . My advice for nonrunners is not to use running shoes. In general, a firmer midsole that one might find in a tennis or volleyball shoe gives better control and the soft midsole is unnecessary anyway." Some of the shoes that are sold specifically for walking (Avia, Reebok, for example) are softer than tennis and volleyball shoes, so generally a court shoe gives more support. Holt continues: "Most walking shoes and even some lightweight hiking boots often have midsoles that are too soft for someone with structural abnormalities. If any shoe has a particularly soft midsole, it can potentially cause problems for the individual with structural abnormalities."

A walking shoe is good for everyday wear unless you are a diabetic and have increased sensitivity to your feet, in which case a running shoe would be better for shock absorption and stability. Walking shoes may also have some of these problems:

◆ Not enough room in the forefoot
◆ Not enough support in the rear foot
◆ Less forefoot cushioning than running shoes

◆ Flexing or bending at the wrong point
◆ Too soft a midsole

In summary, the right shoes make a world of difference and are a quick and highly effective way to sharply decrease your wear and tear and your pain.

9

Restore Your Joints

YOGA

How retro. How sixties. How sort of beatnik-era hip. Or perhaps too New Age? Trust me, yoga may be the single most effective way of dealing with wear and tear or even mild to moderate arthritis.

I learned this from an incredibly enthusiastic young yoga instructor at the Topnotch at Stowe Resort and Spa in Stowe, Vermont. I'd been meaning to commit to yoga but after having looked at several kinds, such as Hatha and Ashtanga yoga, I just hadn't found the right program. The instructor, Cindy, told me that there *was* something new in yoga called Bikram, also known as hot yoga. It was strenuous, athletic, even aerobic. That afternoon I took the class. I wibbled and wobbled, trying not to look like an utter fool in front of the other students. (Fortunately, she banished me from the front of the class.) I struggled and sweated. Then I felt it. Wow! The most perfect stretch I had ever imagined, with a silky smooth feeling flowing through my right thigh. At the end of class, there was this sudden descent into a state of relaxation that I had never experienced before. Amazed, I resolved to go to the Mecca of Bikram yoga, the Yoga College of India in Los Angeles, California. This is the Parris Island boot camp of yoga, the toughest place on the continent. When I arrived, I was sent to the back room. The temperature in the room was 105 degrees. I tried so hard I had to drop my head because of a sudden rush of faintness. Two days later it happened: the pain was gone, the stiffness was gone, the aching hip in the middle of the night was gone. I learned that over time we destroy our bodies. With Bikram, you can restore them. Think about it: we maintain airplanes, cars, even washing machines to counteract daily wear and tear, why not our bodies? Bikram had extended the careers of top athletes by years by restoring their bodies, now it was extending mine! John McEnroe was its poster boy. Bikram allows you to continue playing the hardest of sports, such as tennis or skiing, and then restore yourself in an evening session of Bikram. I found 50 percent or greater increases in range of motion than with any conventional stretching program. You're not just stretching the muscles, you're opening up and restoring the joints.

The conventional wisdom: Stretching is enough.

The real deal: Only yoga will open your joints and restore your youth.

It was after an orthopedic surgeon told me my hip was shot (one too many bike crashes!) that I took the Bikram class. A month later I'd gone from twelve Advils a day to none, gotten rid of all the pain, and increased my flexibility to that of an eighteen-year-old! And poor old Dr. Bob is not alone! Cardiologists from Cedars-Sinai Medical Center, Los Angeles asthma doctors, and chiropractors refer their patients to the Yoga College of India. In 1972, President Richard Nixon was in Hawaii for a summit meeting with Prime Minister Kakuei Tanaka of Japan when he had a severe flare-up of the phlebitis thrombosis he had been suffering in his leg. After treatment failed, the doctors considered amputation of his leg. The decision was made not to amputate for fear of developing gangrene. Bikram Choudhury, the originator of Bikram yoga, was brought in. Bikram treated Nixon for about three weeks with hydropathic treatment in a hot tub with Epsom salts, using movement in the hot water and a full sequence of Bikram's yoga series. Bikram claims he saved Nixon's leg. Richard Nixon became vigorously healthy again.

Take another case, that of a forty-year-old woman I know. I'd watched her stumble up the long set of wrought iron stairs at the local ski area. Her hips and knees were obviously punishing her with every step. Her joints were so stiff, it almost hurt to watch her move. She'd given up the sports she loved, hiking and skiing. Dressed in a leotard, she entered a large room where the temperature was well over 100 degrees. More than thirty men, women, and children drenched in their own sweat, which was literally pouring off their brows, silently followed the directions of what seemed like a drill sergeant's rat-a-tat-tat series of instructions. The only difference between boot camp and this was that boot camp seemed easy by comparison. My friend could barely bend in any direction, and when she did, the pain was almost unbearable. Fast-forward to two months later. The same woman nearly flew up the stairs to the gym, her pain and stiffness gone. Her flexibility was more like that of a teenager. She was free from pain and off her medications. What happened to her? Yoga!

Look at how ancient cultures managed the pain of aging. In a world before Advil and Aleve or aspirin, they found that exercise was the way to do it. Dr. Howard Dananberg, a New Hampshire sports podiatrist, says, "What they did was to develop yoga and tai chi. They developed movement exercises to maintain ranges of motion that allow you to maintain the normal joint mobility. It wasn't lifting tons of weight, it was gentle stretching and gentle mobilization exercises for the joint capsule." Other countries still rely on these ancient methods as the primary means of treating wear and tear—with great success. Bikram Choudhury told me, "When I was living in India, we never heard of wear-and-tear arthritis in India— nothing." And yoga has stood the test of time. Developed over thousands of years, it works perfectly for removing much of the pain of wear and tear. The movement pathways and gentle motions had the bugs worked out of them centuries ago.

When I first asked about how long yoga takes to work, I was

told that it took years! Ugh! I thought, I don't have years! Others likened it to the steady drip of water onto a stone which would eventually change the shape of the stone. That could take centuries! I'm happy to report that the changes occur far more quickly than that! You'll notice the first changes within a week—far faster than most medications take. But unlike medication, yoga keeps on working. The longer you do it, the better you get!

WHY YOGA WORKS

It bears repeating: this has been the single most effective measure I've ever taken to beat wear and tear and restore lost youth. So what does it do?

It provides pain relief. First and foremost, what yoga delivers in spades is pain relief. Unlike medication, which provides episodic relief, yoga offers permanent relief of the aches and pains of wear and tear.

It stabilizes your joints. Dr. Benno Nigg, director of the Human Performance Laboratory at the University of Calgary, is one of the world's foremost biomechanics researchers. I asked him why yoga works so well in cases of arthritis of the hip. He told me that it's the tremendous forces produced by the large muscles that are one of the major contributors to the forces within a joint. The pain in a joint is proportional to the acting forces. He argues that the joint forces (and the resulting pain) are substantially reduced if the *smaller* muscles are used to stabilize a joint.

Others attribute the development of abnormal gait patterns to the loss of fine muscular control of the hip abductors. (The abductors are the muscles that lift your leg to the side.) Yoga strengthens and coordinates the small muscles that exert fine control over our joints and protect them from sudden impact and jarring movements. The best posture for this is called the Awkward Pose, described below.

It's the world's best stretch. I tried to stretch for years but each time

I tried I gave it up. Why? Take the quadriceps stretch. Sure, there was a little tug on the muscle, but I honestly never noticed much difference after I stretched and my flexibility remained close to that of a stone. Yoga delivers a much more dynamic stretch through a far greater range of motion. I went from being able to just touch my ankles to being able to put my hands on the floor. A recent survey of nearly forty-five thousand people showed that as people grow older, the first thing they start cutting out in their workouts is stretching. I know—I'm one of them! To put stretching back into your workout, there's nothing that beats yoga.

It restores your range of motion. Imagine giving up a lung or a kidney. You'd do anything to save one of those vital organs. Yet most Americans are willing to lose half or more of their joints' function by abandoning the joints' natural range of motion. Sound preposterous? Try squatting or sitting cross-legged on the floor. If you can't do it, you've surrendered a large part of your hip and knee range of motion. You'll find that yoga has the remarkable ability to salvage the full use of your joints. What's more, as we've seen, the limitation you find in the range of motion of your knee and hip is very closely linked to the degree of disability you have in that joint. A consistent finding of patients with wear and tear of the knee is decreased range of motion in hip and ankle, as well as the knee.

It repairs your joints. Oh, my aching joints! you may say. But it's not your joints that are aching at all. The joint surfaces themselves don't have pain-sensing nerves. So the pain that you perceive is really around the joint rather than in it. That is, the pain you feel is in muscle, tendons, ligaments, and other parts of the joint. Those are all structures that can be repaired. Most of the pain you feel is from the *secondary* effects of wear and tear of structures around the joint—which is why if you fix those, the pain goes away. Also, since you are improving strength and coordination, you are protecting your joint from further damage. The gentle squeezing and pressure on the cartilage give it the stimulus to repair itself without sharp blows or sudden impact. You're also preventing secondary damage, damage done to your joints because pain and stiffness have forced you to walk awkwardly, exerting harmful forces on your joints. For instance, really tight hamstring muscles can force you to walk with flexed knees. That creates increased and abnormal forces on the joints, says physical therapist Kevin Wilk.

Remember, wear and tear is not merely a disease of articular cartilage but one that involves all of the tissues of the joint, including the bone.

It helps renew your joint surfaces. Excessive contact and pressure between the two opposing surfaces of a joint can worsen arthritis. One reason is that in some patients with arthritis there are calcium crystals, which may become embedded in the joint surface. Yoga pulls those opposing surfaces of the joint apart and away from each other. Alternately, there's an apparent catch-22: too little joint contact pressure fails to provide enough stimulus for the cartilage to repair and renew itself. Yet large shifts in joint contact pressure, which can occur due to faulty biomechanics, also damage cartilage. Yoga is an ideal solution because it stimulates the joint surfaces to renew themselves yet prevents the excessive shearing, tearing, and high-impact forces.

Also, we know that small attachments form within joints that are not fully active. That means that the surfaces that slide back and forth over each other actually start to adhere to one another. In the most severe cases, the joints become immobile. Yoga breaks up these microadhesions little by little.

It helps your balance. Ever wonder how a ballerina can balance on the tips of her toes for seemingly endless periods of time? Practice! That same practice at yoga will give you an uncanny and precise sense of balance you may never have had before. I'm a far better ski racer now than I was in my twenties just because of the balance. Remember, with wear and tear, there is a loss of neurological sensing in the muscles that control joints like the knee. The combination of strength and balance training you get with yoga is a terrific way to repair and restore that lost neurologic function to further protect your joints.

It helps defeat the stiff man syndrome. Yoga resculpts the body beautifully. The stiffness and restrictive movement in your joints are slowly but surely erased. Your posture, range of motion, flexibility, and strength all improve. Over time you'll find you have a new body, one you'll hardly remember from your youth. The hallmark of yoga is gentleness. If you tried to attain the range of motion using other measures, you'd likely injure yourself. Once I tried to increase my hip range of motion on weight-training equipment. One machine in particular was a hip abductor apparatus. I'd sit and see how far I could open up my hips. I'd force them as far apart as possible and then pay the price: I'd have a limp for the next several days! What happened? A structure called an osteophyte on the rim of the joint was limiting the amount I could abduct my hips. My range of motion never improved, and I was left injured!

It spreads the load. The stiff man syndrome that so many of us suffer from restricts our normal range of motion. That can mean excessive and abnormal wear on the joint, especially the hip, since so much force is concentrated on such a small part of the hip joint during everyday activities such as walking. Yoga opens up the joint to restore normal biomechanics and allows the load to be spread over much more of the joint surface.

It builds elasticity. Yoga makes muscles more elastic. That means that for any given load, the muscle can better absorb the shock in a shorter range of motion. Take, as an example normal walking. As you land, more elastic thigh muscles absorb more loads over a shorter distance, better protecting your joint. Yoga is a great overall method for increasing your shock-absorbing capabilities. Joints can also be protected from damaging peak forces by maintaining or improving the compliance of the soft tissue around the joint. That's where yoga helps as well.

It helps build up your feet. As we saw in Chapter 3, feet are the root of much wear and tear. They are also terrific shock absorbers if used properly. Yoga strengthens the arches of the feet, lessening your chance of foot injuries and even stress fractures. I'm always a little fearful of tearing my Achilles tendon. Practitioners of yoga seldom suffer such tears.

It helps conquer stress. Best of all, yoga has got to be the finest way on the planet to *completely* relax! If you can't sit still to meditate passively, you'll find concentrating on a yoga posture the most effective way of taking your mind out of the maze of worries and concerns that plague modern life. Why is decreasing stress important? Stress creates higher levels of hormones such as cortisol and adrenaline. These both dampen the effectiveness of our immune systems.

According to Howard Kent, director of the U.K. charity Yoga for Health Foundation, if stress can cause disease, then "peace and calm can cause health." Dr. Bill Fair, a former cancer surgeon, explained to me during an interview for the NBC Nightly News, "If we put cancer into animals and we stress the animals by a variety of ways, the tumors grow faster. It follows in my mind that maybe if you have a tumor and you destress the animal, the tumor might grow slower. And in this case I was the animal." Dr. Fair was diagnosed with colon cancer. It recurred twice. He hopes that his program of conventional and alternative medicine will help prevent its return. What impact does this have on wear and tear? If you're one of those people whose shoulder and neck muscles tighten during stress, you probably feel that those muscles are getting worn and torn on a daily basis. Yoga is the best way I've found of leaching the pain and misery out of my shoulders and neck.

It's gentle. Many patients with the aches and pains of wear and tear find exercise programs too painful or strenuous and either never get started or quit. Yoga is extremely gentle to the joints. Yoga allows you to chip away at your stiffness inch by inch without pain or strain. Just moving an extra inch and holding a position to the count of twenty is enough to begin improvement.

It builds strength. I took several private lessons with one of Bikram's top instructors. He was cut like a competition-level body builder. He had in fact done years of weight lifting. Now, he told me, he did only Bikram. He maintained the competition-level cut with yoga alone. If you work hard at it, yoga can deliver a complete, highly functional weight-training program.

If it sounds as if yoga is the perfect solution to wear and tear—it certainly can be! If you do nothing else in this book, learn several yoga postures and let them work their quiet magic!

YOUR YOGA PROGRAM

The Postures

Although in America we see yoga as a smorgasbord of postures, in India you are actually prescribed specific postures. I've selected the very best postures there are for highly specific conditions—first to open up the hip, second to restore the knee. These yoga poses are tailored to specific joints and come from the top practitioners of therapeutic yoga. If you have old injuries to your joints or more than moderate arthritis, you may want to review them with your doctor and your yoga instructor. The self-tests in Chapter 2 can direct you to the set of postures most appropriate for you.

A regular routine is terrific for your overall health and conditioning, and that's the way most Americans take it, as part of a class or set routine. Every evening I do the entire set of Bikram poses found in Bikram's excellent book, *Beginning Yoga Classes*.

What you'll see here is a specific set of postures for the hip and knee.

The Science

Part of the problem that alternative medicine faces in the management of many diseases is that conceptually it doesn't fit very well into the double-blind study pattern. "Blind" studies are conducted so that neither the doctor nor the patient knows who is getting the treatment and who is not. Obviously you can't really blind people to the treatment for some types of alternative therapy such as yoga.

More recently, two small studies published in the *Journal of Rheumatology* and the *Journal of the American Medical Association* by Marian Garfinkel and H. Ralph Schumacher found that yoga helps with pain associated with osteoarthritis and carpal tunnel syndrome. Another study at Stanford University showed that yoga was an effective complementary treatment for musculoskeletal diseases like wear-and-tear arthritis, and researchers at the Roosevelt University Stress Institute in Chicago found that "yoga stretches reduced physical stress while increasing physical relaxation." The best existing study on arthritis and yoga studied the hand and was featured in the *Journal of Rheumatology*. Wear-and-tear arthritis can affect the small joints of the hand, the furthest-out joints of the fingers, and the middle knuckle area, particularly in the thumb. Marian Garfinkel and her coauthors raised the question in this study: can yoga improve the outcome?

The researchers measured pain in and function of the hand. They asked about stiffness as well. After a ten-week program, there was another evaluation session comparing how patients felt at that session with the one ten weeks previous. The reduction in hand pain was statistically valid. They also improved range of motion in the hand and that's exactly what you would expect and hope to improve. This is the best-known study and the one most often cited for the benefits of yoga on wear and tear.

WARNINGS

Injuries

The postures here have been selected very carefully for safety. The one complaint I do hear time and again from physiatrists is

that they diagnose a number of back injuries from new yoga afi-
cionados. Dr. Gregory Lutz, chief of physiatry at the Hospital for
Special Surgery, has seen patients who have developed herniated
discs by doing overaggressive yoga exercises. I feel very good about
the safety of the Bikram program. If you do have back problems,
and especially if those problems involve intervertebral discs, be
sure to get your orthopedic surgeon's blessing first! Better still, review the postures with your physical therapist or physiatrist for
their biomechanical soundness. Also, solid programs advise you to
"understand and respect your pain" and teach you to perceive the
difference between the general discomfort of arthritis and the pain
arising from overuse of a joint. Since wear and tear affects different
parts of cartilage in different people, movements that provoke pain
will differ from one person to the next. Pain that lasts more than an
hour after finishing your yoga is a good indication that at least one
posture was too stressful. By learning to understand my pain, I
could distinguish between muscle pain and joint pain. I'd press
hard through the muscle pain but respect the joint pain. You may
also have a substantial amount of irritation in the tissues around
your hips and knees. Press gently through this. My very first yoga
class was a major turnoff. Every joint hurt so much, I was sure I
was damaging my joints. I felt as if I were ninety years old. Over
time, all of that irritation disappeared. Beware of "x-rated" exercises that offer high risks but low rewards, such as the headstand
and shoulder stand.

Also, if you have severe arthritis, have suffered a major injury,
or are over sixty-five, be extremely cautious about beginning a
yoga program. Once a joint becomes badly damaged and highly
immobile, there is a real danger of further injury. For that reason, I
would consider beginning yoga in these circumstances only with
the consent and approval of an excellent physiatrist—that is, a
physician who specializes in joint biomechanics. Slow, careful
range-of-motion exercises supervised by an expert physical therapist are often good if you have severe arthritis or restricted range of

motion. If you decide to take up yoga, you want a teacher who has good credentials.

Joint Laxity

While stiffness can create joint pain and worsen arthritis, the other end of the spectrum may be equally as bad. While you do want to increase muscle range of motion, you don't want to make the joints themselves lax and unstable. Here's an example. Many yoga poses call for a straight leg. In fact, you'll often see participants hyperextend their knee to the point that it almost looks bowed. Experts such as Charles Matcan of Manhattan's Haealth (the spelling is Old English!) Center warn against that.

A straight leg should be just that, neither flexed nor extended. It should be one where the joints are in line with one another. That still gives you lots of leverage to stretch your muscles without overstretching key ligaments that support the knee. I made this mistake big time! The instructor barked, "Straighten your leg!" In an effort to "straighten" my leg, I ended up hyperextending my knee. This created a deep aching pain in both knees. Fortunately, another instructor pointed out that what was needed was a balanced position with the leg straight, supported equally by the quadriceps and hamstrings. He said, "Don't pack it in," meaning don't let the leg collapse into itself in a hyperextended position. "Don't collapse into the joint. Come out of hyper into straight." Good advice!

BREATHING

As a physician, I never believed that breathing differently could have any effect on anything. I now practice deep breathing several times a day to cut stress and instantly reinvigorate myself. Central to all yoga poses are breathing exercises called Pranayama, which can help the spine through their effects on rib movements and pressure within the chest and even abdomen. Many of us, as we get tense, tend to hold our breath in, taking small, strained breaths and stiffening our muscles. Bikram taught me this posture himself.

Directions

1. Stand with your feet together, pointed directly in front of you. Interlace your fingers with your hands raised in front of your chest as if in prayer. Now lift your hands so that your knuckles are directly under your chin. Keep the palms together, again, your knuckles tightly interlaced as if you are praying. Keep your knuckles right under your chin during the entire sequence.

2. Inhale deeply through your nose with your throat constricted just enough to make a noise as you breath in. This acts as a brake to slow your breathing down, which is key to the exercise. Your mouth should remain shut. Inhale in a slow and deliberate fashion to the count of ten. Bikram has a nice way to think about this: "Feel as though your lungs are a glass of water that you are filling from the very bottom up to the rim." This means that you are first feeding air into the bottom of your lungs. As a co-ordinated movement, simultaneously and slowly raise your elbows "like seagull wings" on either side of your body. As your flexibility increases, try to move your elbows higher and higher until they touch your ears. The genius behind the raised elbows is the ability to open up the chest.

3. Now lower your chin but leave your arms in place. Be careful not to bend your entire body forward. As you do, open your mouth slightly and slowly exhale over the count of ten. The first time you do this you may feel slightly short of breath, but as you learn to fill your lungs more and more fully, you'll gain confidence that you have enough air. As you exhale, continue to constrict the back of your throat slightly.

4. As you exhale, drop your head back as far as you comfortably can. Your arms and elbows should rise up and come together as you keep tight contact between your knuckles and chin. Try to gently force every last ounce of air from your lungs.

5. Do a dozen complete cycles, rest, and then repeat another dozen cycles. At the end, drop your arms back to your sides.

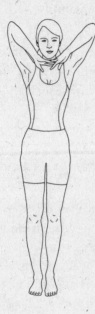 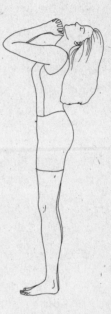

TARGETS

There is an amazing variety of yoga positions you can practice. From a purely practical viewpoint, however, there are very few limitations of movement associated with actual disability. For wear-and-tear arthritis of the hip, we're looking at improving knee flexion, hip extension, and hip abduction. For arthritis of the knee we're targeting knee flexion, hip flexion, hip abduction, and hip external rotation. The therapeutic yoga asanas (poses) we will focus on target primarily those.

The description of each of these postures is for one side of the body. You'll want to complete the mirror image of it on the opposite side of your body, so that you complete a matched set of the exercises on both the left and right sides. Each pair of exercises should be repeated so that you complete a total of four. The phrase "reverse the pose" means that you follow the directions for the pose in reverse to bring yourself back to the beginning stance.

The Hips

These are the poses I've found best aid stiff hips with a limited range of motion and mild to moderate arthritis. The hip has several key patterns of motion that are important to exercise.

1. Proud Warrior (Triangle Pose)

About the Pose

Here's the safest and most gentle way to open up your hips. Why? Because you rely solely on your own muscular strength and not the weight of your body or the mechanical arm of a weight-training machine. Your muscles open and support your hips safely. I tried desperately to open up my hips with weight-training machines such as the hip abductor machine. By "open up," I mean rotating my hip so my foot could turn to the outside by as much as 90 degrees. That led to just more pain and a slight limp. There are no telltale signs that you've pushed too hard with the machine until hours later. What's impressive about this pose is that it opens the hip in two ways: First, there is a straight abduction movement. Second, there is an external rotation.

Basic Directions

1. Stand with your right and left legs about four feet apart.
2. Begin with your hands at your sides, then move them directly away from your sides until they are parallel to the ground, as if you were making a spread eagle. Keep your palms facing downward.

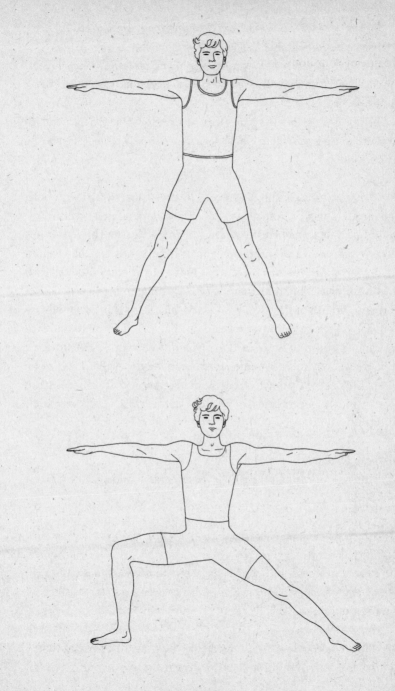

3. Keep your left leg straight, and then point your right foot and leg to the side at a 90-degree angle to your left foot.

4. Point your left foot to your left at a 45-degree angle. Keep an equal amount of weight on both feet at all times, even though you may feel as though you're favoring your right side.

5. Now lower yourself by bending your right knee until the back of your thigh is parallel to the ground. Turn your body so that your belly is brought around to face forward.

Tips: You'll get maximum hip benefit by pressing forward with both hips at all times as you press downward with your left hip. You should be able to feel your right hip opening forward and your left hip opening forward and downward. Concentrate on that feeling in your hips. Breath into them by slowly exhaling as you push into your hips, using the same pattern of breathing and throat constriction you did in the Pranayama. Gently increase your range of motion. This is the safest motion I've found in any exercise to increase hip range of motion without risk or pain. Keep your back straight, even though there is a tendency to lean to the right. Lean your upper body slightly backward. Both feet should stay flat on the floor. You can get terrific hip benefits out of this even if you stick with this basic stance.

Advanced Directions

This is a continuation of the basic stance and picks up from Step 5 above.

6. Lock your arms in the position you've assumed above with them at right angles to your trunk.

7. Bend your upper body to the right. Keep leaning your trunk to the right until your right elbow is directly in front of your right knee and your fingertips are gently touching the floor with your palm facing forward.

Tips: I like to press back with my right elbow against my right knee to further open my right hip. Look upward toward your extended left hand with your chin against your left shoulder. Your arms should form a straight line from your left hand extended overhead to the fingertips of your right hand on the floor.

8. Reverse the pose by straightening your right leg as you bring your upper body to an upright position. Bring your feet together as you drop your arms to your sides.

2. Wind-Removing Pose

About the Pose

Hip flexion deteriorates in all of us as we age, but we rarely notice it unless we test for it. Then one day we discover that a quarter to half our range of motion has just plain disappeared. Although Wind-Removing Pose may conjure up a different image, you'll find it a solid way to regain lost range of motion.

Directions

1. Lie flat on your back with your arms at your sides and your palms facing the ceiling.

2. Pull your right knee up toward your chest by grabbing your leg a couple of inches below your knee with your hands clasped together, fingers intertwined.

3. Now pull your knee as far into your chest as you can. Be sure your left

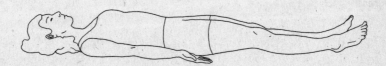

leg remains flat on the ground rather than being pulled off the floor, as is the tendency.

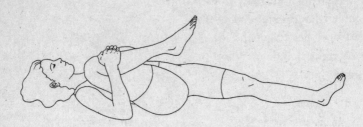

Tips: Relax your feet and shoulders. You may notice a hard stop against which you cannot pull your knee any further into your chest. Nonetheless, continue to pull your knee in slowly but firmly. You should feel a pull in your right hip. Breathe into your hip to extend your range of motion, using the slow Pranayama style. "Pranayama" simply means "breath control." Controlling the breath helps to control the mind. Pranayama is used in yoga as a distinct practice to help clear and cleanse the body and mind. It is also used in preparation for meditation, and in asanas, or poses, to help maximize the benefits of the practice and focus the mind. Press your entire spine into the floor.

4. Now tuck your chin into your chest with your head remaining on the floor. Hold for twenty seconds, then lower your leg to the floor.

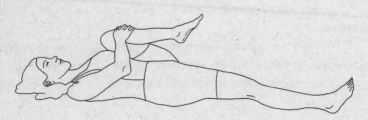

3. Standing Head-to-Knee Pose

About the Pose

We've looked at the importance of the muscles that stabilize your hips. This is the best single exercise I've found to strengthen them. It's also the best hamstring stretch I've found yet. Tight hamstrings limit the amount of rotation you get around your knee. That limits the natural amount of "relief" the knees can get during walking since it blocks a natural part of the knees' range of motion. It's no accident that most people with wear-and-tear arthritis of the knee have very tight hamstrings. Experts find that stretching the hamstrings makes people feel better almost immediately.

Tight hamstrings are linked to back, knee, and hip pain as well. The Standing Head-to-Knee Pose is one of the very best yoga exercises for quickly and effectively releasing your hamstrings.

Basic Directions

1. Place your feet together.

2. Slowly lift your right foot off the ground in front of you.

3. Continue to lift your right knee as high as you can with your leg dangling below it.

4. Cradle your right foot with both hands, your fingers interlinked beneath it. Your index finger should be about an inch back from the ball of your foot.

5. Wrap your thumbs across the top of your toes.

6. Pull your foot up as high as you can, straightening your leg in front of you, to start stretching your hamstrings.

Tips: You'll want to get quite comfortable with your balance so that you can recover quickly if you lose your balance! For the first week or so, this will be the best you can do. Some yoga masters ask you to actually bow your standing leg. Other experts would rather you simply keep it straight. I prefer the straight leg if you have any signs of wear and tear, to prevent any joint laxity. In either case, don't progress to the advanced directions until you can get the bend out of your standing knee and come to a completely straight position.

Advanced Directions

7. Straighten your right leg out in front of you with your hands still cupping your right foot. Your right leg should be parallel to the floor.

8. Bend your trunk forward until you can touch your forehead to your knee. Hug your leg with your arms and elbows. To keep your balance, fix your eyes on a single point on the ground.

9. Push your heel forward, away from your body as you pull your toes toward you. Both legs should be straight.

10. Reverse the pose slowly and straighten up.

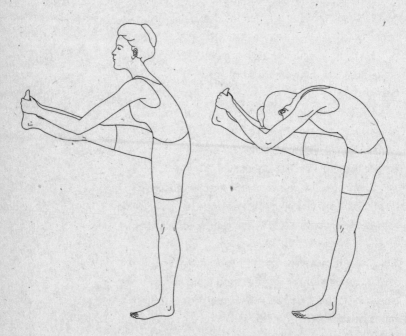

Tips: In reality, it may take weeks to months until you can completely straighten your leg, but you're still getting lots of benefit just by straightening it to the point where you feel a burn in your hamstring.

4. Head-to-Knee Stretching Pose

About the Pose

This is an exceptionally rewarding yet easy pose. It's a gentle but highly effective way of opening up your hips. You can apply leverage to your hips in small, safe increments. This is also one of the finest back and hamstring stretches.

Directions

1. Sit on the floor with your right leg and left legs flat on the floor and out to the sides, each at 45 degrees from the centerline. Try to form a 90-degree angle between the two legs.

2. Pull your left heel directly into your groin, knee bent and dropping to the outside. Try to bring your heel as far up your right leg as possible with your forefoot against the inner part of your right thigh. With time, you may be able to drive your left knee flat onto the floor. Early on, your left knee may still be well off the ground.

3. Grab your right foot with your hands cupped, fingers interlaced under the ball of your foot and your thumbs. This will give you maximal leverage for the next step. You'll find it a very comfortable fit.

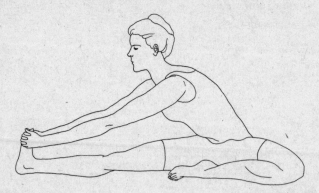

4. Pull your right forefoot toward you, keeping your right leg straight with the back of your knee on the floor. Stretch your upper body directly down over your right leg.

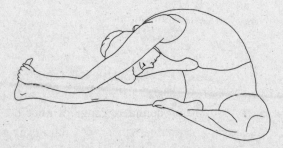

Tips: As you lower your upper body, point your elbows toward the floor. Try to touch your forehead to your knee, tucking your chin into your chest. I still can't do this part, but over the last several months I've been able to get my left knee closer and closer to the ground. Remember, the stiffer you are, the more exercise you're getting because you have to put in more effort!

5. Stay down at least to the count of twenty and then slowly come back up to a sitting position as you bring your left leg back to a resting position on the floor.

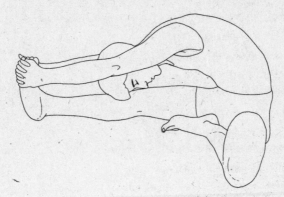

The Knees

These are the exercises I've tried and found to be the most effective for the knee. Bikram agrees that most of the problems are in the quadriceps muscle, limiting range of motion and causing tightness, so most of the exercises are directed at the quadriceps.

1. Awkward Chair

About the Pose

This is a real standout for bad knees. I'll admit that the first time I tried the Awkward Chair, it didn't seem humanly possible, but I was able to regain my complete range of knee flexion and strenghten the small stabilizing muscles protecting my hips and knees.

Another common flexibility problem of knee patients is that the ankles can become very tight because of the way they stand and walk. In fact, a consistent finding in patients with arthritis of the knee is decreased range of motion of the hips and ankles, as well as the knee. The Awkward Chair will help increase the range of motion of the hip, knee, and ankle. There are three separate parts to the Awkward Chair, each with its own separate stance. They're included as part of one exercise because you do need to move directly from one stance to the next.

Directions

Part 1

1. Stand with your feet and knees six inches apart with your feet parallel to each other.

2. Raise your arms directly in front of you until they are parallel with the floor.

3. Keep your palms down and your fingers together with your arms six inches apart.

4. Concentrate on a single point directly in front of you and keep your gaze focused on it.

5. Sit down as if there were a chair behind you until your thighs are parallel with the floor.

Tips: Keep your heels flat on the floor. Exhale as you check to make certain that it is the backs of your thighs that have lowered themselves into a parallel position with the floor and stop there. Don't be disappointed if it takes several weeks until you can get all the way down. Try to keep your hands from rising as you sit. Keep your muscles firm.

6. Roll your weight back onto your heels while you try to straighten your back as much as possible. Be careful not to fall over backward when you first try this. Get your back into a position as if it were up against a wall. Start by arching your back. Let your weight roll onto your heels, lifting your toes. Stay down for at least the count of ten.

7. Come up as slowly as you came down. Keep your feet, arms, and hands all six inches apart and your hands parallel to the ground. Stand up on your toes like a ballerina.

Part 2

1. Bend your knees as you lower yourself halfway toward a squat.

2. As you descend, force yourself up onto the balls of your feet, pressing your heels higher and higher into the air to get further onto your toes. You should have a nicely arched foot with your heels as high and as far forward as you can press them. Your spine should be as straight as possible.

3. Continue to lower yourself until the backs of your thighs are again parallel to the ground. You'll think this is an almost impossible art of balance when you start. But with persistence, you will succeed! Stay down for a count of at least ten. Bikram would encourage you to press higher and further forward with your heels each time.

4. Slowly come up to a standing position, allowing your heels to sink back to the floor. Keep your arms up, straight, and parallel to the floor.

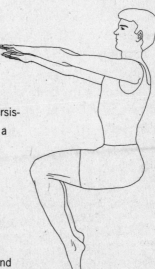

Part 3

1. Place your feet six inches apart and rise up on your toes a little bit.

2. Bring your knees together so the insides are touching.

3. Keeping your knees together, bend them and lower your buttocks toward your heels. Come up slightly on your toes as you're descending.

4. Your thighs should come to a rest in a position parallel to the floor, as should your arms. Your spine should be at right angles to your thighs. Try to keep your arms from rising up from their parallel position. Stay down for a count of ten. Return to a standing position.

Tip: You may not come anywhere close to bringing your buttocks to your heels in the first months of performing this pose. You'll still reap lots of benefits even if you don't. Be sure that you control your movements with your thigh muscles at all times.

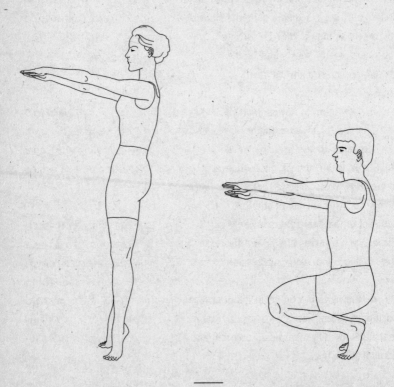

2. Eagle Pose

About the Pose

The Eagle Pose looked so daunting, I thought it impossible—at least for the first month I tried it. The idea of wrapping one leg around the other seemed ludicrous. I could barely get one leg to touch the other!

Yet you'll find the Eagle Pose one of the best measures of your progress. This pose is a great way to build balance, coordination, and strength in your legs. The pose also helps you develop the fine muscular control that will protect your knees and hips. This pose develops amazing balance. If you're like me, you'll think that the fine sense of balance to stop from falling over is beyond reach. However, by using fine rapid movements of your foot and ankle and by developing an acute position sense in your foot, you'll get there faster than you imagine. The Eagle Pose is one of the niftiest and most biomechanically efficient ways of doing a one-legged squat I've found.

Directions

1. Stand with your feet together.

2. Intertwine your arms as best you can in the following fashion. Place your left arm straight out in front of you. Now place your right arm underneath it with your right elbow crossing just above your left elbow (above meaning your upper arm). Bring your right hand toward your face as you twist your right arm around your left. Try now to place your palms together.

Tips: Don't be disappointed if you're a long way off when you start. Over time, try to get so you can interlock your fingers as if saying a prayer. Your thumbs should face your nose as you bring them toward your chest. If your shoulders are riding up, try to lower them by pulling down as hard as you can with your arms. Bikram told me this is a great way to relieve tension from the neck and shoulders. Try it next time you're stuck waiting to go through airport security!

3. Wrap one leg around the other in the following fashion. With your feet together and your back straight, bend both knees about six inches. As you're bending your right knee, lift your right foot up as high as your left knee. This is the point where you're going to wrap your right leg around your left. Bring your right foot across the front of your left knee and then behind it. By bringing your right foot up high, you'll create the momentum you need to lower your right foot into position behind your left calf.

4. Once your right foot is behind your left leg, hook the toes of your right foot behind your left leg around the lower part of your left calf muscle. I try to "crawl" with my right toes to pull my right foot into position.

5. In the third part of this terrific pose, you'll basically do a one-legged squat. Here goes! Keep your back straight and both hips facing forward. Sink as deeply as you can into a one-legged squat, aiming for a 90-degree angle between your upper and lower legs. Try to stay down for at least ten seconds. You do want to press your legs together firmly. Slowly come back up as you untwist your legs and arms.

Tips: If you're really wobbly, you can untwist your arms and use them for balance in your first week. Focus and concentrate your gaze sharply on one point in front of you to prevent losing your balance. Concentrate on your feet too. Big movements from your knee up may topple you. Fine foot and ankle movements are the key! Don't be afraid to use a wall to catch yourself during the first

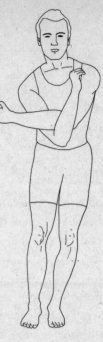

week. This is one of the toughest poses, so don't be concerned if you get only halfway there!

3. Standing Bow-Pulling Pose (Dancer's Pose)

About the Pose

This is the finest single quadriceps stretch on the planet, in my view. Tight quads can pull on your kneecap and increase pain when running, cycling, skiing, playing tennis, or exercising on a stair machine. Several recent studies have documented that patients with wear and tear of the kneecap have tightness of the quadriceps. The Standing Bow functionally lengthens your quads up to several inches, thereby relieving the pain and allowing you to continue to play. Why? There's less tension in the quads, less to pull on your kneecap. The Standing Bow-Pulling Pose also helps to extend the hip to increase the functional range of that joint.

Directions

1. Stand balancing on your left foot alone. Shift your weight slightly forward onto the ball of your foot so you can feel the shift in weight across the forward part of your foot to react quickly. Some weight should remain on your heel.

2. Put your left hand straight up in the air above your head. Place your right hand by your side.

3. Press both arms backward to get as much stretch as you can.

4. Rotate your right hand so the palm is facing outward with your thumb pointing toward the back.

5. Lift your right foot directly behind you while bending your knee. Try to get your foot as close to your buttocks as possible.

6. Grab the instep of your right foot with your right hand. The key is that your wrist should be on the inside of the foot, not the outside. Hold your foot just below the ball of your foot with the sole of your foot facing the ceiling. This will seem awkward at first but is brilliant in concept, delivering much greater leverage than the traditional quad stretch.

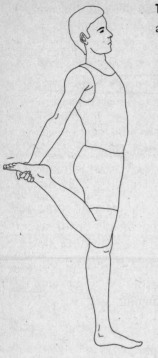

Tips: Keep both arms close to your body and avoid rotating your foot out to the side. Your standing leg should be straight and not bent. Avoid overextending your left leg. Keep your left hand overhead.

7. Press your entire torso forward so it looks like an archery bow. Push forward hard with your hips so that there is a smooth bow in your body from your chest through your right hip to your right knee.

8. Bikram describes the final step better than I can: "In one solid piece from hip joint to fingertips, roll forward like a wheel until your abdomen is parallel to the floor. At the same time, point your toes and kick your right foot upward and backward with all your strength, straining against your cupped hand."

9. To maintain your balance, fix your gaze on a single spot on the wall in front of you. Be sure your hand doesn't slip.

Tips: When staring straight into a mirror, you should see one foot appear to come out of the back of your head. Keep pulling your foot higher over your head. You should get a very strong pull on the hamstring of your standing foot. It's important to concentrate on pointing down with your hip. This doubles the amount of stretch you'll get in your quads. You should feel a good firm stretch through your chest, abdominal, hip, and quad muscles. Don't be afraid to have a wall nearby the first couple of times you perform the Standing Bow-Pulling Pose.

10. Hold for 20 seconds, then slowly return to an upright position.

General Tips

There's a tremendous amount to be learned from the right yoga teacher. They can quickly fine-tune each pose. Viewing tapes or reading books can get you 90 percent of the way there, but consulting an expert can help you get the most out of each pose. Here are some tips I've collected from expert yoga instructors:

1. Toes are reachers and feelers, *not* grippers. Use your toes for position sense and try to spread them as far apart as you can, rather than using them like a claw to hold on.

2. Don't make things worse in an effort to make them better. If you're too aggressive in your efforts to turn back the clock, you may hurt yourself. For instance, I've tried very aggressively to open up my hips, only to find myself hobbling for several days afterward. I've found that pressing firmly against muscular resistance and pressing through the tightness is highly effective. But pressing through real pain, when you're pressing bone against bone, can have poor results.

3. Breathing is the heart of yoga. In everyday life we hold on to excess tension in our muscles, especially our neck and upper backs. Even while undertaking yoga postures, there may still be excess tension in muscles that hold you back from achieving the perfect posture. Develop good breathing habits, and you'll cut tension in your day-to-day life and improve your success with yoga.

4. Don't pack your joints! This is an expression experienced yoga teachers use. What it means is that you want to avoid "collapsing" into your joints. Here's an example. During a hamstring stretch there's a natural tendency to hyperextend your knee. That can cause joint laxity. If you keep your leg straight without allowing it to hyperextend, you get all the stretching benefits without placing your knee at risk. So come out of the hyperextended position into a straight-legged position.

5. Find your weakest link. Stress goes right to your weakest link. That's where you'll feel pain and tension every day. Find your weakest link and strengthen it to cut the effects of stress. For many of us, it's the muscles in our neck or back. Dampen stress by relaxing and invigorating the muscles that it hits the hardest.

6. Develop a "foot sense" in the standing position so that you are keenly aware of where the pressure is on individual parts of your foot.

Yoga is making a major comeback. Although it may seem the latest fad, it's a medicinal art thousands of years old that can have remarkable effects on real patients with real diseases. The scientific literature shows that yoga can improve conditions from asthma and bronchitis to arthritis and diabetes. Blood sugar levels are improved in diabetics and functional breathing capacity in asthmatics. In countries such as India, where the majority of the population cannot get medical care from doctors, they often rely on yoga for therapy—and it works!

This slow, deep breathing isn't just good for asthma; it's amazing for cutting the effects of stress and pushing into areas of soreness. What's more, yoga was developed, some say, as a gentle way to ease the body into old age with the grace and suppleness of a teenager.

10

Build Protective Strength

M agic bullets! They're the stuff dreams are made of in the American public's fascination with medicine. Pharmaceuticals powerful enough to cure a dangerous or disabling illness. There is no such wonder drug for wear and tear. But there is something far more powerful in its ability to dramatically reduce your pain and disability. It's strength!

The conventional wisdom: I'll wait for the cure.
The real deal: Bodily strength beats anything in a bottle.

Maximizing the strength of the surrounding muscle takes the load off the joint. This decreases the rate of acceleration of joint degeneration. There's another even more fascinating reason. Exercise improves the quality of the joint fluid so that the joint gains improved shock-absorbing abilities. After twelve weeks of strengthening exercises for the quadriceps muscle, researchers found that the viscosity of the joint fluid increased, as did the molecular weight of its most important shock-absorbing component, hyaluron. Strengthening the muscle can also tighten up the ligaments that support the knee, decreasing excessive side-to-side movements and thereby decreasing irritation to the joint.

When you look at the benefits of strength training compared

to medication as a way of reducing pain, the rewards are tremendous, according to Colonel Gail Deyle, chief of physical therapy at Brooke Army Medical Center at Fort Sam Houston in San Antonio, Texas. First, the cost of medication, which can run to thousands of dollars per year, is saved. Second, the treatment of bleeding ulcers is avoided. And third, joint replacement may be avoided.

BEGINNING EXERCISES

If on the tests in Chapter 4 you found yourself quite weak, here are two easy exercises you can do at home. They're recommended by Sharon Feldmann, physical therapist and clinical manager of the Arthritis Center at the Rehabilitation Institute of Chicago. If you passed the tests in Chapter 4 easily, skip over this section to the advanced section.

1. The Yellow Pages

Choose a phone book about three inches thick. Stand with both feet on the phone book. It's a good idea to do this next to the kitchen counter or a steady table to use for balance and support. Now, start by lowering yourself and stepping forward off the book with one foot, always leaving the other foot on the book. The leg that you are standing on is the leg that is being exercised, not the leg that is stepping down.

Make sure you bend your knee as you do it. One common mistake is moving your hip instead of your knee. Make sure you know what your knee is doing by looking at yourself in a mirror. Pointing your leg slightly to the outside will help to recruit hip stabilizers and buttocks muscles as you descend and helps you maintain alignment. This makes the stress on the knee more symmetrical and doesn't put pressure on the inside. As you lower yourself, go slowly. This is vital to gaining maximum benefit. A slow, controlled motion works your muscles best in this exercise. Repeat five to ten times with the left leg followed by five to ten with the right leg. This will build endurance. Try to do three sets of five to ten repetitions with each leg. By alternating legs you can exercise continuously through the three sets. As you improve, you can increase the height of the object. As an example, use the bottom stair of a staircase. In terms of the activities of daily living, stair climbing is pretty much at the top of the list, as is the ability to get out of a chair. This exercise will help with both.

Here are some tips for descending a staircase: Keep your knees over your toes. Don't let your knees turn in, which is the most common error. Going down the stairs is the same idea as this step-down exercise; you want to make sure to control your descent with knee flexion rather than simply dropping your hip. When ascending stairs, be sure to lean forward a little bit. Many people lean back instead and push off with the railing.

2. The Beer Run

The first twelve minutes of *Law and Order* have finished. The commercial break is long enough to get up and grab a complete meal: Miller Lite, Doritos, pretzels, and cheese puffs. You push down into the sofa and launch for the kitchen. But wait a minute! Next time, keep your hands off the sofa or chair. With good form, use your buttocks muscles to rise out of the sofa. If you can't do that without pain (it's actually easier and less stressful if your seat is higher), add a cushion to adjust the height. Work on standing up and lowering back down into the chair with good alignment and control—don't just fall back into the chair. Here's the best form, as suggested by Sharon Feldmann.

1. Scoot forward until you are at the edge of the seat.
2. Get the feet under the knees.
3. Lean forward at the waist, so that you are in the best mechanical position to just push up and have your legs do all the work. It's your buttocks and thighs that are working the most.

Try to do twelve repetitions each time you get up. Eventually lower the seat as your strength improves.

ADVANCED TRAINING

If you had average or better strength on the tests in Chapter 4, the following four exercises will be highly effective methods of improving your strength. In choosing among them, there is one technical consideration.

CLOSED-CHAIN EXERCISES

Academic experts conclude that "closed-chain" exercises are more beneficial, translating your strength to real-world usage and limiting your risk. Classic closed-chain exercises are leg presses and squatting, as well as stair stepping. By "closed chain," physiologists mean your foot is in contact with the ground as an anchor and you employ multiple joints: ankle, hip, and knee. A now-classic study at the Mayo Clinic found the shearing forces between the upper and lower leg were "greatly reduced with closed chain."

The classic open-chain exercise is a knee extension on a machine. Here the foot is not attached to the ground and the chain of muscular involvement remains open. Also, just a single joint is used, the knee, rather than the hip and ankle as well. Experts say this is a less realistic exercise because in daily activities and sports we don't use just one joint. Researchers at Ball State found that "single-joint exercises like knee extensions help strengthen the quads but do little for integrated movements and balance."

1. The Squat

Ugh! Just the name of it conjures up images of high school gym class and sweat-stained clothes. I avoided them for years. However, the squat is the king of leg-strengthening exercises. The squat, quite simply, is the best single exercise there is for building overall leg strength. The squat is the fundamental exercise of choice.

It's the foundation of countless exercises performed to enhance strength, coordination, and function, says Eric Greeno, physical therapist and team leader at the Rehabilitation and Sports Medicine Center at Florida Hospital Celebration Health.

Safety The safest squats are performed as part of yoga postures, because these postures have been perfected over thousands of years.

The squat uses all of the major leg muscles in the buttocks, thighs, and calves. When you sink a little over halfway down, the hamstrings get their biggest workout. The quadriceps and calf muscles peak out when you sink all the way down to 90 degrees. That's important, because the maximum benefit is derived from lowering yourself to that 90-degree angle, when your upper leg forms a right angle with your lower leg and your thigh is nearly parallel to the ground. That doesn't mean you have to start with this full range of motion. Try beginning with a minisquat, which will bring you about halfway down to about a 45-degree angle.

Colonel Gail Deyle suggests an assisted minisquat if you're unable to squat on your own. Rest your arms on parallel bars in a gym or on two chairs, one on either side of you at home or the office. Squat to about 40 degrees or until you feel the first tightness in your knees or calves, then push yourself up to standing using the muscles in the front of the thigh and the back of the hip (quadriceps and gluteals). Keep those muscles tightened for three to five seconds after returning to the upright position. The arms may be used for balance or a slight assist as required. By using these hip and thigh muscles to return to the standing position, they also push against any tightness in tissues limiting the full upright position of either the hip or the knee.

Colonel Deyle determined in a study published in the *Annals of Internal Medicine* in February 2000 that a combination of manual physical therapy and clinical exercise in combination with a home exercise program resulted in 52 percent improvement in pain, stiffness, and functional ability in patients with wear-and-tear knee arthritis. Colonel Deyle emphasizes that all the exercise and manual treatment techniques used in his study either were painless or produced minimal symptoms that abated quickly after the session. Patients were taught to exercise in the same manner during the clinical and home sessions.

Another way to ease your way into doing squats is to slide down against a wall. You can also put a therapy ball between you and the wall. As you improve, add resistance by adding bands, a barbell, dumbbells, or a partner. The squat can be performed with two legs or one leg, on a flat or uneven surface. It can also be performed on a machine called the Smith Machine, where the range of motion is fixed.

Essentially, the number of ways you can perform the squat or its variations is limitless.

Form The key to a safe, effective squat is what's called a hip-dominant strategy, sticking your butt backward. The basic squat is performed using only your body weight.

Directions Start with your feet shoulder width apart. Your feet can be pointed forward or slightly outward, allowing you to engage more muscle for a greater benefit. Lower your body by bending your hips and knees. Pretend that you are sitting in a chair placed a little behind you. Pay special attention to specific body parts. Keep your head up. Tighten your stomach. Hold your arms and hands straight out in front of you to help counterbalance your movement. So both legs get a good workout, try not to lean away from your weaker leg. As you descend you should still be able to see the tips of your toes. Descend only to a point where your thigh is parallel with the floor and your lower leg is roughly at a right angle with your upper leg. If you shift your weight too far forward over your toes, your knee may experience excessive shearing and compressive forces. Rise back up from a deep squat in the same coordinated fashion. Be sure to keep looking forward with your head up and back flat to slightly arched. Your hands can return to your sides. Repeat until your muscles fatigue. To build strength, perform more repetitions or add weights, with the assistance of a trainer.

Warning As you squat, your kneecaps receive a progressively greater load because your body weight shifts forward toward the

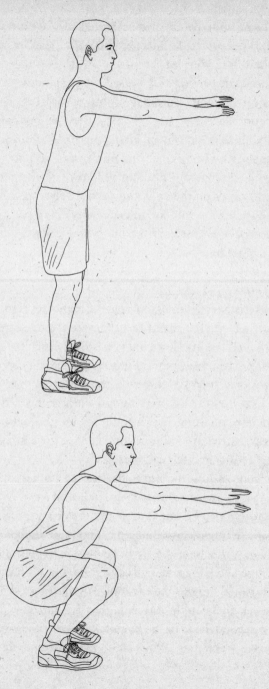

joint surfaces underneath them. A squat also tightens and compresses the knee joints. The deeper you sink, the more compressive force there is until your leg is bent at a 90-degree angle. In physical therapy circles the word "arc" is used. For instance a physical therapist may restrict you to a range of 0 to 60 degrees. Those 60 degrees of motion are the "arc." If you suffer kneecap pain there are two ways to beat this problem. First, you can do minisquats, which limit your squat to between 45 and 60 degrees. Second, performing a squat while sliding your back up and down against a wall can be a good deal easier on the knee and produce significantly less pain. Dr. Neil Roth adds, "I'm not an enormous fan of squats because I think they load the kneecap a lot, but [with] low weight or even no weight [they're] fine."

2. The Leg Press

Most resistance-training equipment manufacturers produce a leg press machine. The majority of these are used seated, and the exercise is directed in a horizontal position. Since the leg press is performed horizontally, there is less weight-bearing force, making the compressive forces less during the leg press than during the squat. This makes the leg press a good exercise to start with if you have difficulty squatting. Work your way up to squats after developing greater strength and function. The leg press strengthens the buttocks, hamstrings, and calf muscles.

Directions Adjust the seat to the desired amount of knee bend. Physical therapists, after reviewing studies of knee rehabilitation patients, recommend beginning at the lower knee angles at first. That means setting the machine up for no more than 60 degrees of flexion. This is the "safe zone" where most activities of daily living are performed. The leg press places minimal stress on the kneecap in this functional range. One advantage of the leg press is that when the stress is highest on the kneecap, that pressure is widely distributed over the underside of the kneecap, making it less painful than a knee extension exercise. You can build into deeper flexion angles of about 100 degrees, where electrical traces show there is more activity in the quads.

Place as much of your foot on the footpad as possible and grasp the handles by your seat. Your head should be erect. Use a wide stance with your feet slightly turned out. The wider stance gives you a bigger base of support, better balance, and easier movement. Turning your feet out brings the buttocks muscles more into play when doing a leg press, which is easier on the knee, is less demanding, and allows for more balance. Dr. William Kraemer adds that some pieces of equipment for the leg press take the lordosis out of the lower back and create more shear forces at the back and knees than any other exercise. So machines have to be used carefully, as some are better than others. While comfort at the starting position may be of help, if you are put out of the anatomical position, it can be bad.

Movement In a controlled manner, push the pedals out until the knees and hips are completely extended. It is not necessary to lock the knees when the legs are straight. Then, in a controlled manner, return to the starting position. Your back and head should remain against the backrest at all times.

Safety Be careful that your feet don't slip off the pedals. This can easily occur when only the toes or balls of the feet are placed on the pedals.

Number of Repetitions Start with eight to twelve repetitions. Your weight should be high enough that your muscles fail on the last repetition. This should work out to about 75 percent of the total amount of weight you could lift just once. Since that percentage is notoriously hard to work out, experts such as Dr. Kraemer recommend staying within this eight- to twelve-rep training zone. Repeat three or four times in each workout. After your strength has improved you may reach a plateau in your training. This often occurs after about six weeks. At this point consider alternating your workouts each week with a light, a moderate, and a heavy day:

- **Light day:** Twelve to fifteen reps with light weight, repeated three or four times.
- **Moderate day:** Eight to ten reps with moderate weight, repeated three or four times.
- **Heavy day:** Three to five reps with heavier weight, repeated three or four times. These heavy reps are important even for older people, Dr. Kraemer says, because "certain tissue isn't recruited unless you lift heavy weights." This is the one set in which you don't want to go to failure because of the extra compression on the kneecap.

The recommended sequence is heavy on Monday, light on Wednesday, and moderate on Friday.

Warning On the leg press machine, the forces are pretty low, from about 0 to 60 degrees. From 60 degrees and beyond they dramatically increase. The deeper you go, the higher the forces are on your kneecap.

3. Knee Extension

Directions Sit on the knee extension machine with your knees just over the edge of the seat. Adjust the seat so your spine is touching the back of the seat. Adjust the footpads so that the fronts of your ankles are touching the footpads. Grasp the seat or handles provided. To begin with, adjust the machine so that your knee is at a 90-degree angle, which is the position it will naturally assume if your lower leg is dangling over the edge of the seat. In a controlled manner, straighten your knee until it's at a 40-degree angle or about halfway extended. Hold for two seconds. This is the most tolerable range of motion. Then in a controlled manner return to the starting position. Don't use your upper body in an attempt to help straighten the knees. Use only the front of your thighs to perform the exercise. Work your way up to higher angles of extension only if the exercise remains pain free. Dr. Kraemer says: "You need to be very careful when doing full-range-of-motion ones compared to, say, thirty-degree arcs as ripping the heavier weight loads off the stack can exacerbate knee problems and stress the knee joints."

Safety Avoid unnecessary jerking movements, especially of the lower back, since this may cause injury. This may occur if you try to lift too much weight. You may also need to place padding behind your back if it doesn't touch the back of the seat.

"The leg extension has really gotten a bad rap as the culprit of many knee problems," notes physical therapist Kevin Wilk. "I don't think it's bad as long as you keep the weight low, you move up gradually, and you're doing the proper angles based on your type of pathology." If you have pain, either lighten the load or stop the exercise.

Warning The knee extension can be very painful in full extension because the greatest amount of pressure is put on the smallest area of contact on the undersurface of the kneecap in this position. This in turn might explain why patients with knee arthritis experience pain during leg extensions. The greatest load occurs as you move your leg through the last part of the exercise into full extension. For this reason, physical therapists recommend a "limited arc" of motion. This "limited arc" of motion should be pain free. Start at 90 degrees so that your thigh and lower leg are at right angles. Then extend your knee only 30 degrees to the horizontal, stop, and return your leg to the starting position, suggests Tim Stump, M.S., PT, CSCS. By avoiding full extension, you cut the stress on your kneecap substantially. Recent literature suggests that doing knee extensions from 90 to 30 degrees is relatively safe, says Mark Reinking, physical therapist and assistant professor at Saint Louis University.

4. Standing Dead Lift

Having very strong quadriceps and weak hamstrings can set you up for an injury. Dr. William Kraemer recommends dead lifts as a simple, at-home way of strengthening the hamstrings.

Preparation Place a barbell on the floor. Your feet should be shoulder width apart or less, and you should arch your back by sticking out your buttocks. Bend at the waist and grip the bar with your hands about shoulder width apart.

Starting Position The knees should be slightly bent as you lift the bar off the floor so it's close to the shins. Keep your back straight and your shoulders pulled back. You should look up, which helps to keep the back in the appropriate position.

Movement Now contract your hamstrings and gluteal muscles, while straightening from the hips to bring the weights up. Although there is lower back involvement in this exercise, the drive should come mainly from the contraction of your hamstrings and gluteals. When you first begin to do this exercise, begin with a very light weight (e.g., 10 pounds), and concentrate on feeling the sensation of squeezing your hams and gluteals.

Safety Be sure not to round your back and pull your shoulders forward. Of utmost importance, never lock the knees when doing this exercise. Be sure to check with your doctor first.

HOW TO PROTECT YOUR JOINTS DURING TRAINING

Strength training can be a double-edged sword. On the one hand, you're creating the power to protect your joints. On the other hand, there is a real risk that you will injure yourself or cause overuse that will worsen your symptoms. To avoid that, I've put together these tips from leading experts:

♦ Look for machines that work the way the human body does. These are called ergonometrically correct machines. Brands such as Cybex and Hammerstrength are carefully designed to take into account the natural biomechanical patterns of the body. Poorly designed machines may hurt your knees from the very first repetition. There are only a handful of machines designed by engineers who understand human biomechanics. You may also find that a machine can't adjust to your body's dimensions. The most important example is a knee extension machine. Some of these may not line up with the axes of your knees. That places undue strain on your knees and is certain to hurt. Often certified physical trainers at the gym can show you how to use the equipment properly.

◆ Take your time working through the whole range of motion of a joint. You may start by using just 20 degrees of the joint's natural range of motion during your first week. Over weeks to months gradually increase your knee range of motion to 90 degrees.

◆ Be very careful using the full range of motion with leg press machines. There is a tendency to pull your knees almost up to your chest and then explode into full leg extension. This puts tremendous compressive forces on your lower back. Even with a low weight you can end up with a herniated disc. Be sure your lower back does not come off the machine. Secure your lower back by placing a towel between the small of your back and the machine. This prevents excessive flattening.

◆ Avoid overload. Using the same machine with the same weights week in week out can cause a condition called pattern overload. You can avoid this by changing the machines or exercises you use and varying the amount of weight. This is called "periodization." A trainer can help you set up a schedule that has you train with light loads one week, medium loads another, and heavy loads a third.

◆ No pain, no injury! "Push through the pain" is a common exhortation by physical trainers. If you have muscle pain, pushing through does bring you to a greater level of strength. But if the pain is in your joints, chances are you are doing more damage. In my own program, I built up the range of motion and strength first with yoga, then with weight-training machines. With yoga, pushing through muscle pain is a great deal safer.

◆ Develop your coordination. We've talked a good deal about the coordinated use of muscular strength. For instance, if you are thrown off balance walking over rough ground, you could injure a joint. That means you need not just strength but coordination. You'll get that by using balance platforms, one-legged yoga postures, and free weights.

HIP STABILITY

We haven't talked much about the hip muscles, yet they're incredibly important in terms of protecting you against wear and tear. Here's why. When you transfer all of your body weight to one leg, you use two sets of muscles. In order for you to keep your leg aligned and keep your pelvis level and not drop it down, your hip abductors and extensors hold you in position. But if they're weak, then every time you step on that leg, one of many things can happen. For instance, your pelvis drops down, your leg turns in, your knee turns in, or both. This places abnormal mechanical stress on your hip and knee joints. If your pelvis drops down, you're overstretching the abductors, which makes them weaker. The abductors are the muscles that move your leg outward to the side. There is one yoga posture that builds strong abductors: the Standing Head-to-Knee Pose. You'll find it described on page 147.

SLOW TRAINING

Weight training at very slow speeds has been all the rage for several years. Gary Hunter of the University of Alabama found that the traditional workout burned about 50 percent more energy than the super- or ultraslow training. The reason? "Simply because you can't use any weight. Anything that you can do ten seconds up and twelve seconds down and eight to twelve reps has to be incredibly light. We found that nobody could handle any more than 25 percent of his or her maximum weight, and that's incredibly low weight. We also measured metabolism when they were doing it, and it was very, very low. This certainly wouldn't be good for increasing power but probably good for muscular endurance." Hunter points to a new study in the *Journal of Strength and Conditioning Research* that confirms that traditional weight-training procedures also produce more strength gains than superslow training.

WHAT'S THE EVIDENCE THAT STRENGTH TRAINING WORKS?

A key paper in the *Annals of Internal Medicine* evaluated the effectiveness of physical therapy programs and supervised exercise. The researchers found that subjects "experienced clinically and statistically significant improvements in self-perceptions of pain, stiffness, and functional ability and the distance walked in 6 minutes." They also had decreased dysfunction and stiffness. But the most important aspect is that treatment actually deferred or decreased the need for surgery! Strength *is* a magic bullet for arthritis. If you have limited time and can't get to the gym, squats alone can deliver the power, endurance, and strength you need to protect your joints and relieve your pain. Many of us view strength training as a daunting, complicated, never ending avocation. In this chapter we have narrowed the choices down to a small number of beneficial exercises that can be completed quickly and effectively in a limited period of time. Trust me, they'll make a world of difference in the way you feel.

11

Put Back the Spring

Francesco Moser was one of the world's greatest cyclists. *Cycling Weekly* described him in 1987 as "the outstanding Italian professional of his generation—a great athlete who always rode with superb showmanship and panache that kept the fans happy for 14 years." Francesco added more than a kilometer to the ultimate record in cycling—the one-hour record, exceeding fifty-one kilometers—by using the latest in technology from exhaustive wind tunnel tests to an extensive use of sports science. For one week—and a thousand dollars—I joined a dozen club racers for the privilege of training with the great Moser in Florida. On our first morning together, Francesco did not immediately impress us as a great athlete. He was not huge like a linebacker or tall like a basketball player. He was a very average sized man. He did, however, have extraordinarily well sculpted quadriceps muscles. Still, there was something very odd about his quads. In the late afternoon, our entire group underwent therapeutic massages. And that's where the difference became apparent. When the masseuse kneaded Francesco's thigh, she could almost lift the muscle off the bone. It was so supple, so elastic; it was as if he were a cartoon character. We red-blooded Americans, on the other hand, had thighs as hard as rock. The masseuse nearly required a chisel to begin a halfway decent massage. Francesco was so intent on keeping his muscles supple that he refused to run. He even shunned walking for more than a few yards for fear of tightening his quads.

What, you're probably asking, does this have to do with performance? We discovered what the following day during a hundred-mile training ride. At the beginning of the ride, we all spun out of the gate near an impressive 110 revolutions per minute.

Compare that to the average weekend cyclist who manages 50 rpm. That tremendous cadence shows fresh, supple muscles. However, as each ensuing hour approached, our cadence would fall: 100—90—80—70—60. By the end of the ride, we were lugging through the gears with legs as heavy as lead. But Francesco's hour-by-hour cadence was 110—110—110—110—110, a testament to the stunning elasticity in his legs. As the coup de grâce, at the end of the last lap of the last mile, with the rest of us huffing and puffing, frothing and spitting, Francesco briefly stood out of his seat and literally walked away from the pack at a dazzling pace—with the panache his fans had loved him for.

Look at Mark Spitz. Among the seven gold medals he won in 1972 was a gold in the 100-meter butterfly. His time in 1972 was 54.27 seconds. Nearly twenty years later, in 1991, he still completed the 100-meter butterfly in less than a minute, 58.03 seconds. Cal Ripkin never missed a game in seventeen big-league seasons, playing 2,632 consecutive games and breaking Lou Gehrig's 2,130-game streak.

John McEnroe played in the Davis Cup at age thirty-three and on the Champions Tour until he was almost forty in the 1998–99 season.

All of these athletes had elastic muscle capable of producing instantaneous power. Each of them stayed on top of their game years later than physiologists thought possible by maintaining the explosive power that is characteristic of elastic muscle. You may say, Hey, those guys were professional athletes! Indeed they were. I cite them as acid tests. If they can maintain near-world-class performance into their forties, there's great hope for the rest of us.

The conventional wisdom: Muscle should be hard as a rock.

The real deal: Muscle should be soft and pliable. Elastic muscle is youth.

Contrast these athletes' elastic muscle to stiff muscle. A stiff muscle provides tremendous resistance and gives little. That is, there is little change in the muscles length in response to a load applied to it. So, say your heel strikes the ground during normal gait. As your foot lands, your quadriceps pick up the load. A very stiff quad will give little. Stiffness, or loss of muscle extensibility, has been implicated in injury. A very elastic quad will give, reducing the force applied to your joints and providing substantial protection. Elasticity is one of the most overlooked muscle qualities. It's also the newest and on the cutting edge of training. Simply put, when your muscle encounters a force, the stiffer it is, the less of a shock absorber it is. The more elastic it is, the more it protects you. Do you notice, for instance, after a long run or hike, that the following day, you don't just feel stiff, but it actually hurts when you walk? That's because you've temporarily lost a major component of shock absorption.

"In my opinion, the loss of flexibility as we get older is one of the most significant declines in functional capacity. It becomes more and more important as we get older," says James Graves, Ph.D., professor in the Exercise Science Department at Syracuse University. That loss of flexibility and agility is what makes many of us feel old. The spring goes from our step. The acceleration and punch when playing tennis or kickball or even playing with our kids are lost. But the great good news is that you *can* put it back. Aerobics are the basis of most personal-training programs. But the repetitive motion of walking, running, or hiking slowly steals our elasticity. With just a few basic exercises you can put it back.

If you have moderate to advanced arthritis, there is a risk that you could injure yourself. If you have arthritis or are recovering from injury, you'll only want to consider these exercises with an experienced physical therapist and then only when you're ready. "They are not the safest and probably something you wouldn't recommend for older adults. And probably something you would avoid at least initially in patients with arthritis," says Dr. Graves. The safest and easiest way to begin building elasticity is with cycling. At a high cadence and light load, you'll have a safe and effective way to begin. Over time, as you train at higher power settings and develop the spin of a professional cyclist, you'll find extraordinary explosiveness and elasticity returns. However, cycling doesn't give you the explosive power needed to lift your body weight in athletic sports such as basketball or tennis. For that you'll require an exercise called a "plyo," short for "plyometrics." I'd advise consulting a trainer to be sure you have enough power, strength, and flexibility to begin a program of plyometrics.

PLYOMETRICS

Plyometrics are exercises that are designed to specifically train the eccentric contraction (lengthening) phase of a muscle's work. Plyometrics enable the muscle to reach maximum strength in the shortest time possible. You can think of plyometrics as stretching the body like a rubber band, then contracting back very quickly. The most effective way of building elasticity is with plyometrics. "Plyos," as they are affectionately known, combine speed and strength to deliver power. "Plyometrics are extremely effective at developing high levels of muscular power, which is the ability to exert force quickly," says Dr. Graves. As we saw in Chapter 2, as you age, your muscle is "scarring down" and your tendons are losing their snap and elasticity. Plyos are the final step in reversing the process of scarring down.

Most athletic movements prestretch the muscle to deliver more power. Plyos are also common in everyday activities, such as going down stairs. It's this principle of prestretch upon which plyos are based. Let's take a closer look. Say you're jumping up and down on a diving board. As you land on the springboard, the first part of your power for the next jump into the air comes from the stretch reflex. Receptors in the muscle detect rapid motion within the muscle as you land on the board. These receptors excite the alpha motor neurons, which then command your muscles to produce power. The more it is excited, the more force your muscle can deliver, because you've increased the electrical activity of the muscle. You'll also gain power by stretching the tendons, which anchor your muscles to your bones. For years, researchers believed that most of the elasticity was in the muscle. Now they are convinced that most elasticity is in the tendon.

"Tendons need to be very elastic, as do their connecting points to muscle, because these structures take most of the trauma of daily wear and tear. If you jump up, for example, your tendon, which surrounds and supports your kneecap, will take up a lot of the stress. The more elastic you are, the better it is able to absorb those stresses," says Dr. Vijay Vad.

Here's an example of how a plyo works. Stand on a foot-high bench. (Try this only when your trainer, physical therapist, or doctor says you're ready.) Now drop off the bench with both feet. As you land, try to stop yourself quickly. If you can lock your thigh muscles as you land, the force will stretch your tendons and muscles, like stretching a rubber band. If you time it properly from the point at which you stop descending and lock your muscles, the elastic energy stored in your muscles can be used to lunge back into the air. The key is first having very strong muscles so that you can stop them very quickly, as you are going down, and lock them very quickly.

LUNGES

The Basic Lunge

The lunge was made famous in cinema by the motion made by fencers as they drive toward their opponent. The lunge appears very athletic and beyond the range of many people with wear and tear. However, the lunge is often prescribed in physical therapy clinics, even for arthritis, because of the large arc of motion involved and the many muscles used. Kevin Wilk uses the lunge frequently with his patients.

Directions Take a large step forward with one leg. Now bend the lead leg at the knee until your back knee touches the floor. Check the position of your lead leg. The knee should be over the ball of your foot. As Dr. William Kraemer notes, if your knee is in front of the ball of your foot, your step was not long enough, and as a result you put unnecessary torque on your knee. If your knee is behind the ball of your foot, either your step was too long or you are not low enough. Now here's the key: as you sink down to the floor, you'll want to store elastic energy in your quads and then use that energy to push off the floor with your lead leg. Be sure your back stays straight throughout. As you become stronger, load up your quadriceps with a faster sinking motion onto your quadriceps and explode upward more vigorously. The key is timing so that the lunge becomes one motion. That means melding the sinking action directly into your spring back up. When you begin doing a lunge, have a friend or trainer spot you and help you correct your form. Another tip from Kevin Wilk: "As you lunge forward, make sure the back leg is relatively straight, with just a slight bend so that most of your weight is on your front." Most people try to lunge while keeping equal weight on both legs. What you want is the majority of your weight, 80 to 90 percent, on the front leg. Bend a little bit at your hips as well as in your trunk.

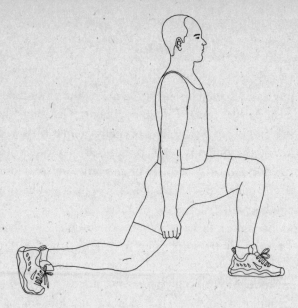

The Two-Step Lunge

The easiest part of the lunge is when you sink into the lunge position. The risky part is coming back up. For many people, the load on the kneecap is just too great. They suffer pain or even injury and abandon the technique. What goes wrong? Pushing back up with one step is just too much load for the tendon that holds the kneecap in place. That's where the two-step technique comes into play.

Directions Sink down as deeply as you can into the lunge position. You should feel a good burn in your quadriceps. Then take two small steps back with your front leg to return to your starting position. Choose any speed you like. Even in rehabilitation the lunge is gaining respectability as a way of becoming more dynamic as you regain functional ability.

The Dumbbell Lunge

Bodybuilders perform lunges with a barbell over their shoulders. This requires significant skill and strength. It also requires at least one spotter. A far safer and easier alternative if you want to add weights is to use dumbbells. You'll also find it easier to keep your back straight.

Directions Hold a dumbbell in each hand with your arms hanging at your sides. The starting and finishing position and the movement are the same as for the regular lunge.

When I first started the program to beat wear and tear, lunges were impossible for me. Pain, stiffness, lack of coordination, and muscular weakness all interfered. Now I love the lunge. The explosive power I've gained goes a long way toward getting those one or two points per game against my eldest son in tennis.

12

Lighten the Load

E ver notice the strained gait of an overweight person who is suffering from wear and tear? You might imagine that that defect would be hard to correct without surgery. Now research has shown that weight loss alone is enough to cause significant biomechanical improvements in gait. Since many researchers see wear-and-tear arthritis as a biomechanical disease, it's extraordinary to see the actual mechanics of walking correct themselves after weight loss.

The conventional wisdom: A few extra pounds won't hurt.
The real deal: Every pound counts.

Patients in a Wake Forest University study reported significant improvements in their degree of disability, knee pain intensity, and even physical performance measures after undergoing a diet and exercise program or even an exercise program alone. Those who both dieted and exercised lost an average of 18.8 pounds! This study was the first to show that older, obese adults with wear-and-tear knee arthritis are capable of losing a large amount of weight. Although obesity has been shown to worsen knee arthritis, the results of this study showed that losing weight can help treat the arthritis after it appears.

This study was the first step in finding out how exercise and diet affect arthritis.

WHAT YOU CAN DO NOW

What's the best approach?

That's far from settled, as evidenced by dozens of different diets and hundreds of books. While you and your physician may want to choose one that is best for you, there are some tips you may consider that could help you with the diet of your choice.

Eat foods that help you lose weight. If you let foods do the job for you, you'll find weight loss a lot easier. While dieting is never fun, there is a large reward in the form of vastly diminished pain.

SATIATING FOODS

These are foods that fill you up and keep you feeling full. Although nutritionists emphasize that the time it takes to feel full is critical, researchers say the length of time you *stay* feeling full is even more important. When I come back from a long trip, I always have a few extra pounds to lose. I do what millions of people around the world do, rely on a grain-and-bean meal combination. This provides 95 percent of all your minerals, vitamins, protein, fat, and carbohydrate. But it provides something far more important: the ability to feel satisfied and stay that way for hours. Why? Beans are the best source of soluble fiber. This fiber provides tremendous long-lasting satiation. Soluble fiber also helps even out and lower your blood sugar and cholesterol levels. The sugar is especially important because by lowering your blood sugar levels, you lower your insulin level—and it is insulin that makes and keeps many of us fat.

Ours is a nation that is overstimulated by food. According to a review of thirty-nine studies in the *Psychological Bulletin,* one factor that's contributing to the overconsumption and increase in obesity is "dietary variety"; that is, foods of different colors, flavors, and shapes. That leads us to the next concept, the "dull diet"!

THE DULL DIET

That's right, one of the best ways of killing your appetite is a dull diet! What do I mean by dull? If you eat foods that have very similar qualities, you become satiated early and stay satiated longer. You've satisfied the taste you expected to satisfy. Now let's say that you're offered a piece of chocolate cake, bacon, or eggs Benedict, and a steak with hollandaise sauce. Could you eat them? You bet. Could you eat all of them? You bet! Why? You've piqued your brain's interest by introducing new tastes and smells that have not been satiated. In fact, your poor brain had forgotten about being hungry until you presented your new food choices. That's because the brain has specific senses to satisfy. If you take one sense and satiate it, you'll feel full—until you introduce a new taste or smell sensation. That's why buffets are such a disaster. When I want to lose weight, I eat highly satiating meals, but the same meals day in, day out. If I'm offered a slice of bacon or a piece of candy, I might end up eating the whole pound of bacon or a whole bag of Rollos. I protect myself by being certain that I *am* full!

Here's a case in point. A classic study by Barbara Rolls invited two groups to a four-course meal. The courses were:

A plate of sausages
A plate of bread and butter
A plate of bananas
A chocolate dessert

One group was given all four courses. The other was also given four courses, but all four had to be the same, e.g., they might have had four courses of chocolate dessert. It is important to note that food's palatability is lessened the more you eat of it. Now here's what happened. The group consuming the four different courses ate 44 percent more food and 60 percent more calories! The sight, smell, and taste of a new food group stimulated the appetite so they could eat far more food than they needed to. This is sensory-specific satiety at its best. How do you make use of this to lose weight? Make sure each meal has similar sensory characteristics. That is, if each food has roughly the same texture, color, and even taste, you will automatically limit what you eat. Here's an example:

Dinner
    White chicken breast
    White beans
    Cauliflower

This is a very satisfying dinner. You'll find you feel full at the end. You'll probably find it so dull you won't eat the whole thing.

The trouble is that we are exposed to such a huge variety of foods every day that there is no natural break that tells us to stop eating. A "cafeteria" diet presents a serious case of "my eyes being larger than my stomach."

Confronted with salad bars, cafeterias, and fast-food joints, we're just powerless to stop eating when we should. The more variety, the more you're likely to eat.

I can't resist, and I know few people who have the willpower to do so. Putting yourself into the wrong situations, such as dinner at a pasta bar, promotes overeating.

I take dull eating a step further and have the same dull breakfast and lunch every day. It cuts down on the time I spend deciding what to eat. Go ahead and have a meal you like. Just regulate the sensory experiences by limiting the tastes and textures as you see in these meals.

Enjoy your selection, but let the limited food choice work for you in keeping your weight under control. This is a kind of behavioral therapy—but it's a whole lot simpler than having to use real willpower! There are many useful tools to help control your weight, and decreasing the variety of your foods is one of them.

The "dull diet" may not be a runaway best-seller—but it'll sure help you fight the battle of the bulge.

HIGH-FIBER FOODS

High-fiber foods are among the most satiating ones. Fiber slows the transit of food through the digestive system, makes you feel full longer, and slows the absorption of fats and sugar. I use them as a fabulous way to kill my appetite and feel full for hours longer than I would with low-fiber food. Studies have shown that people who follow this type of diet reduce their risk of developing heart disease, some forms of cancer, stroke, and diabetes. Donald Corle of the National Cancer Institute reports that those who ate a high-fiber diet consistently over four years gained "greater confidence in their ability to care for their health, greater belief that food choices would improve health, and more awareness of health and nutrition messages." But here's the part I like best: "Contrary to common perceptions of low-fat diets, participants did not report any detrimental effects of the eating plan on taste, cost, the convenience of shopping for and preparing foods, their overall health assessment and general well-being, or satisfaction with life," Corle reported in the August 2001 issue of the *Annals of Behavioral Medicine.*

LOW GLUCOSE LOAD

This is the hottest concept in nutrition today. In study after study, a high glucose load is what puts you at highest risk for diabetes and obesity. This is even truer for women than men. Each day your body is challenged by the amount of carbohydrates you eat. Those carbohydrates come in different qualities, judged by their ability to elevate your blood sugar level. Once you add up all those carbohydrates at the end of the day—and their individual abilities to elevate your blood sugar—you can calculate your glucose load. Foods such as white bread, bagels, and cinnamon buns have a very high potential to elevate your blood sugar. Pastas, rice, cereal, and potatoes have an intermediate ability to elevate your blood sugar. But here's the surprise: if you eat many foods with this intermediate ability, you can still end up with a high glucose load. So if during a day you had a serving each of white rice, boiled potatoes, a bagel, pancakes, and a corn muffin, you'd have a high glucose load. The key is to bring your glucose load as low as possible. I do this by eating only carbohydrates with the lowest potential for raising blood sugar. Those are, quite simply, beans, vegetables, and many fruits. If you were to not eat any carbohydrates with a medium or high potential for raising your blood sugar, you could lose five to ten pounds without a serious attempt at dieting. The appendix has three tables for carbohydrates at low, medium, and high glucose loads.

Why is glucose load so important? Your body responds to a high blood sugar level by producing more of the hormone insulin. Insulin is what then helps store the excess sugar. Excess insulin helps us get fat and stay fat. In theory, a high blood sugar level speeds the aging process by reacting with proteins by forming cross-links, which "toughen" tissues, causing skin to lose elasticity and blood vessels to thicken. This same cross-linking may also occur in tendons and joints, aging them prematurely.

What about fats? Saturated fats are the most important kind of fat to reduce in your diet. The body doesn't need them, and they may actually aggravate arthritis. Fish oils and olive oil are the best and healthiest fats.

PROTEIN

The most satiating food is a pure protein. A famous Vermont prison study asked prisoners to overeat. They could easily overeat carbohydrate or fat but underate protein. Think of it yourself. Can you eat a couple of bowls of pasta? Sure! What about several servings of french fries? No problem! But try to eat four swordfish steaks. Or take the challenge of a famous steakhouse in Texas: if you can eat a fifty-ounce steak, it's free. The chances are high that you'll fail. To use this strategy to your advantage, begin a meal with protein, which will kill your appetite early in the meal. I always start with protein to kill my hunger and steady my blood sugar level. When I really want to strip off the pounds, I'll have an all-protein breakfast and lunch. It makes me mentally sharp as a tack, drops my glucose level dramatically, and kills my hunger. I then make sure to get my vegetables in the afternoon and evening.

SAMPLE MENUS

Here are a day's sample menus. You'll see how protein always comes first in a meal. When I want to lose fat quickly and effectively, I'll begin each meal with protein and then eat only fruits and vegetables.

There is also a sort of salvation factor. What's that? That means that as you lose the weight, exercise becomes easier, you can move around more, and you then acquire a synergy that gets the weight coming off faster.

BREAKFAST

Menu 1
    Soy milk
    Very-high-fiber breakfast cereal, for example, Kellogg's
        All-bran
    Cantaloupe

Menu 2
    Huevos rancheros: scrambled eggs made with egg whites with
        beans on a whole-wheat tortilla

I had this breakfast one morning in Aspen before a three-hour climb on my mountain bike. I literally was not hungry again until nightfall. Since then, if I really want to lose weight, I'll have this breakfast, take a long bike ride, and watch the pounds melt off!

LUNCH

A big piece of chicken or fish
or
One Boca burger
or
A bowl of vegetarian chili
or
A bowl of spicy black bean soup

EARLY DINNER

One black bean and wild rice burrito made with a whole-wheat tortilla, in the proportion of three quarters rice to one quarter beans.

SNACKS

At home, have just one snack food available rather than stockpiling doodles, chips, and pretzels. Even better, choose a healthy one. You're far less likely to overindulge, for instance, on blue corn tortilla chips or Scandinavian Bran Crispbread, a product of Norway.

For more meal plans and recipes, see my cookbook, *The Breast Health Cookbook* which includes healthy meals for both women and men.

HEALTHY FAST FOODS

These are commercially available meals and dishes that can be prepared quickly in a microwave.

Cascade Farms: These are my favorite meals in a bag. They have a great mix of veggies, beans, and healthy grains. They're enormously satisfying meals that will keep you full for hours. They're ingeniously designed to be tasty. My favorite meal is the Aztec Vegetarian Meal.

Fantastic Foods; Nile Foods: These are meals in a cup. Add boiling water or put into the microwave and you have a highly satisfying and filling meal. I like the black bean soups, which can deliver up to 17 grams of fiber!

Boca Foods: Boca burgers gained fame as the vegetarian burger of choice in the Clinton White House. They're quick to microwave or grill and taste terrific. I love the breakfast patties, which taste like pork sausages but are made with soy.

Boutique soups: Soups can be surprisingly great meals. Good soups combine high-fiber beans, large amounts of antioxidants, and phytochemicals. For those of us too rushed to buy, prepare, and cook five veggies a day, a soup can be a great all-around meal that does all the work for you. If you're going organic, which can be time-consuming and expensive to do on your own, consider Walnut Acres. I like their Mediterranean Lentil Soup.

13

Play Joint-Friendly Sports

DATELINE: HOKKAIDO

Mike Mosher is one of NBC's most brilliant foreign news produc-
ers. For days we had tried to get within spitting distance of a volcano threatening the Japanese island of Hokkaido. The area had
been cordoned off by the military and was closed to the world press
corps. The aggressive Japanese press had tried without any success
at all. Then Mike hit on a daring strategy: we would ride with the
Japanese defense forces! Hours later we were at the base of a road
that would take us directly to the volcano. The military let us park
at the base of the road to get a shot, then they left us. We could
hardly believe our good fortune. Wow! We could see the volcano
spitting lava and belching smoke. Mike, the cameraman, the sound
man, and I started to walk up the road. With helicopters buzzing
overhead, we were just positive that we were going to get nailed for
entering a forbidden zone. Each time the helicopters came within
range, we hid under a tree. After several hours of cloak-and-dagger
work, we closed in on a small forest. The cameraman captured
spectacular pictures from within a hundred feet of the nearest lava
bombs. As the sun set, we made our way back down to our vehicle.
But the closer we got, the more my hip hurt. It seemed to seize up.

Our total distance wasn't more than a few miles. What had gone wrong?

The big surprise to me was that, as I learned later from experts, walking can cause a striking amount of pain and even damage. You may say, Gee, walking is supposed to be good for you. You're right, in part. Sure, there's aerobic benefit. And it can be good for the cartilage as well, stimulating it through compression. But if your joints are already damaged, if the way you walk is imperfect, if you have fatal flaws in your skeleton, you may quickly accelerate the damage to your joints.

The conventional wisdom: I have to cut back on the sports.
The real deal: Hammer away—but at a joint-friendly sport.

Dr. Joseph Feinberg, physiatrist at the Hospital for Special Surgery in New York City, lays out the dilemma: "First of all, it's true if you have an arthritic joint and you continue to load it, you're going to further traumatize it. But if you have an arthritic joint and you *don't* use it, it's going to stiffen and you are going to lose function. So to me, it's more important to maintain mobility and function than it is to limit the arthritic process."

The solution? The good news is that there are joint-friendly sports. This chapter is a treasure trove of them.

Dr. Feinberg says that ideally you want to perform exercises that promote joint motion while minimizing significant loading. For arthritic knees, Dr. Feinberg says that stationary cycling is ideal, but other exercises, such as the StairMaster, elliptical trainer, and NordicTrack, load the knee joint, but to a lesser extent than the treadmill does.

The final test of just how friendly they are to your joints is to give them a try. For instance, I swear by stair machines, whereas some other people complain bitterly that they kill their knees. Many casual observers look at elite-class runners and shake their heads, imagining the terrible consequences: banged-up knees and broken-down hips. On the contrary, elite-class runners have the least evidence of arthritis. "Long-distance runners have been studied more than any other type of athlete, but despite the repetitive stress to their feet and legs, runners who train for many years do not appear to be at increased risk," says David Nieman, Ph.D., professor of health and exercise science at Appalachian State University in Boone, North Carolina. In fact, Professor Benno Nigg, director of the Human Performance Laboratory at the University of Calgary, found that those with the very highest impact loading rate had the lowest risk. "Why? Part is natural selection. Elite runners have perfect biomechanics, very low body weight, amazing shock absorption, and no fatal skeletal flaws."

The truth is, there is no such thing as a bad sport. So this chapter will look at the sports that produce the smallest amount of twisting, sharp impact, and high loads. Which works best for you will depend on your own biomechanics, as described in Chapter 3. If you have certain fatal flaws, running and walking could still be the worst thing you can do. But don't feel you have to abandon a sport you love. I like the strategy of Dr. David Krebs: Don't feel you have to give up a sport entirely. If you get knee pain playing tennis, stop for a few days or a week. Go to the pool, get on your bike—or do some weight work, then gradually get back into it.

AEROBIC EXERCISE

With so much emphasis on weight training, yoga, diet, and weight loss, aerobic exercise often gets short shrift in a program to beat wear and tear—especially since many aerobic exercises can worsen wear and tear. The usual doctrine about aerobic exercise sounds worn and old. Sure, it increases muscle strength, speeds weight loss, improves mobility, and enhances well-being. That's nothing to sneeze at, but here's the real crown jewel: the most alluring reason to undertake aerobic exercise is that it may have a direct beneficial effect on your cartilage.

◆ In hamsters that ran on a wheel, there was greater production of a key component of cartilage called "proteoglycan" and less damage to the cartilage.

◆ In humans, physical activity creates increased cartilage thickness.

◆ Then there's the reduction in pain: patients with hip or knee osteoarthritis who walked three times a week actually decreased their pain.

◆ Dr. Marian Minor, Ph.D., PT, and associate professor in physical therapy at the School of Health Professions at the University of Missouri, looked at patients with rheumatoid arthritis who had swollen joints. She determined that after they did aerobic exercises, swelling went down by almost 50 percent.

◆ A study was done comparing walking and cycling to isometric exercise. Scientists were actually able to measure blood flow in the joint lining, called the synovium. What they found was that those who walked and biked had better circulation than those who did the isometric knee exercise that we traditionally had assumed was the best thing to do for a swollen knee. They also found that when the knee was held in a bent (flexed) position, the circulation actually decreased.

JOINT-FRIENDLY SPORTS

These sports will all give you a good workout while going easy on your joints.

Bicycling

My bike has been one of my best friends for years. Why? First look at the advantages. No matter how much you weigh, once you're seated on a bike, your weight is neutralized. But here's why I like cycling best. I can put out tremendous amounts of power without loading up my joints. How is this possible? In a simple word, cadence. By spinning the crank arms at a high number of revolutions per minute, each individual stroke carries a low load, while the overall power output is high. Think of yourself as a Ferrari in first gear with your tachometer pegged at 6,000 rpm. There's just no other sport that allows you to create that kind of power with your legs without placing huge stresses on your hips and knees.

Kevin Wilk agrees: "The bicycle is easy on the joints and very good from a resistance standpoint." Mickey Levinson, physical therapist at the Hospital for Special Surgery, echoes, "Biking is probably the best because it has lesser load" on the joints.

The bike can also cause very positive changes around the knee even if the bike's resistance is set to zero! That's right. Even if you set the load to zero, you're decreasing the stiffness around your joints. "What I was really looking at (in my recent study) was the cardiovascular responses and so these people all had aerobic training effects and they had decreased pain," says Kathleen Mangione, Ph.D., PT of Arcadia University. Patients with arthritis often find that they rapidly decondition, meaning that the aerobic power of their heart and lungs quickly diminishes. The great news is that they can gain that back very easily by cycling. A recumbent bike with a chairlike seat is easiest of all for those who are infirm. My father had a great deal of difficulty walking, due in part to wear-and-tear arthritis in his hip. Yet cycling was a terrific way for him to remain conditioned. In Dr. Mangione's study, even those undertaking low-intensity exercise found improvement "in the timed chair rise, in the six-minute walk test, in the range of walking speeds, in the amount of overall pain relief, and in aerobic capacity."

A beginner may want to ride ten minutes at a time, three times a week, and increase that by five minutes each week. Another good piece of advice is to buy a comfortable seat. If you're using a stationary bike in a gym, buy a gel-pad-filled saddle cover. For your own bike, consider high-tech seats, which are designed to better accommodate the human anatomy. As you increase your speed, look at the dramatic increase in calories burned per hour, as shown in the cycling chart below. As you become better conditioned, you'll burn an amazing number of calories.

CYCLING CHART

Miles per Hour	Calories Burned per Hour
<10	272
10	408
12	544
14	680
16	816
17	952
20	1,088

Following are some tips to help you get the most out of cycling:

◆ **Use proper equipment.** The first goal is finding equipment that places the lowest load on your knee joint. That means getting a lightweight bike with high pressure, low-resistance tires and great gearing. I use a Litespeed Titanium Road bike with high-pressure tubular tires capable of holding 120 pounds of air pressure. I bought Criserium SSLs, which ride like greased lightning. If you buy a clunker, you'll put unnecessary strain on your joints and also miss out on substantial training benefits. A hefty, poorly geared bike with heavy wheels and high-resistance tires will severely limit how hard you can go before you start putting too much strain on your joints.

◆ **Make sure your cleats are properly aligned.** Many cyclists use a click-in system to hold their shoes on the pedal. These cleats are screwed into the bottom of the shoe. Be sure these are properly aligned, as improper alignment can damage your knees.

◆ **Maintain the correct cadence.** Be aware that you can put huge loads on your knee and even damage them during cycling. I see it all the time in Central Park, really big guys standing up on their pedals and trying to clobber them, putting huge loads on their joints. Why? They're cycling at a low cadence and very high load.

A high cadence is considered to be 90 to 120 rpm. A low ca-dence is below 60 rpm. You can measure your cadence on a computerized exercise bike at the health club or buy a measuring device for your own bike for less than $100. Or you can simply hold one hand above your knee and count every time your knee comes up and taps your hand (this is one revolution of the pedals). Do this for a fifteen-second count and multiply it by four. This is your cadence. Try this experiment. Start at a very fast cadence, say 110 rpm. Feel where the pressure is in your leg. It should be right in the middle of your thigh. Now slow your cadence down. Drop it to 100, then 80, then 60, then 40. This is best done on an exercise bike at the gym, where you can see your actual cadence on a computer readout. Notice how the part of the muscle you are using moves closer and closer to your knee joint. There will be more and more pressure inside the joint itself as your cadence decreases.

Now, you may be frustrated, thinking you're not burning many calories or that you are not developing very much power. Well, cycling has two other huge advantages. One is that you can go nearly forever—honest! The first time out, you'd be sore, but you could go twenty, even forty miles. Try doing that running! Even though cycling feels easier at a higher cadence, you're going faster, getting stronger, and burning more calories.

◆ **Get your weight off your knees.** Climb with your butt. Your largest muscles are the gluteal muscles in your butt. Make an effort when you climb to apply pressure with your buttocks by keeping a low posture and sticking out your butt. I find it much easier on the knees.

◆ **Keep your seat high.** If you have kneecap pain, you may have some difficulty on a bicycle. Put your seat up as high as you can tolerate it so that your leg is in full extension. That uses the part of your knee's natural range of motion that puts the least stress on your knee. This decreases the amount of knee flexion. Dr. Kathleen Mangione concurs: "The seat should be as high as possible but so that cyclers can still reach the pedal when the leg is in the fully extended position. Their knee can be almost completely straight when they are at the downstroke, the lowest part of the downstroke." In a study of elders she found that a higher seat "really limited the amount of bending, which decreased the compressive forces at the knee."

◆ **Consider using a stationary bike.** Dr. Gregory Lutz confirms that stationary cycling is effective and safe for people who have joint limitations, but certain modifications, he says, have to be made in seat position and height. This gentle low-impact conditioning exercise is usually well tolerated, particularly by patients with hip arthritis. Choosing the right kind of stationary cycle that goes along with your joint limitation is important. With some you don't need to bend your knees as much; with others you don't need to bend your ankles as much. Another advantage of the stationary bike is that you can cycle backward. Researchers at the VA Palo Alto Health Care System looked at the effects of backward cycling. They found that it was good for patients with wear-and-tear arthritis and damage to the meniscus because it decreased the compressive forces within the joint. However, cycling backward increases the compressive forces for patients with kneecap pain and injuries to the anterior cruciate ligament. Upright stationary bikes may increase the pressure on your back. If this happens to you, consider using a recumbent or reclining bike, which allows you to sit down in a real seat with a back and take the pressure off your spine. When choosing a stationary bike for your home, look for bikes with proper ergonometrics; that is, bikes that accommodate best the way the human body really works. The best ride silky smooth and lure you back to use them again. The worst have such high resistance at the beginning of the stroke cycle that you'll soon be in pain!

Tai Chi

Tai chi is a moving form of yoga and meditation that includes a number of forms that are made up of sequences of movements. Many of the movements come from the martial arts. Researchers concluded that following just two one-hour classes per week over twelve weeks, participants "experienced significant improvements in self-efficacy for arthritis symptoms, total arthritis self-efficacy, level of tension, and satisfaction with general health status." Little wonder! Tai chi was developed as a way of easing one's way through the aging process. Like yoga, it's been tried over millennia, with fabulous results. I like it best for its ability to build strength. Other functional outcomes that improved included one-leg standing balance, fifty-foot walking speed, and time to rise from a chair. Be careful with tai chi, however, if you have severe arthritis or are over sixty-five.

Yoga

If you're going to do only one activity, yoga should be it. See Chapter 9.

Cross-Country Skiing

Cross-country skiing offers a silky-smooth ride for your joints. I raced the eighty-six-kilometer Väsalöppet in Sweden one year. At the end of the race I felt I could have skied back to the start. There are two different styles of cross-country skiing: striding and skating. Try both to see what's kindest to your joints.

It's worth investing in lessons to learn proper technique. Even after years of racing, I was crushed to learn I'd been skating improperly. I'd smash my ski into the snow, then twist my leg as hard as I could to get onto the next uphill skating strike. Wrong! said Andrew, a fabulous Aussie skier from the Royal Gorge Cross Country ski area, who corrected my form. He pointed out that the more lightly you place your ski on the snow, the more speed you retain. Why? Because you create very little friction. With decent form and well-waxed skis you'll find cross-country skiing is the single best exercise for building up the aerobic capacity of your entire body—and the gentlest on your body! Exercise physiologists call it the "queen of aerobic sports" for good reason. The highest aerobic capacities ever measured were in cross-country skiers.

Water Sports/Aerobics

Swimming is extremely kind to the joints of your lower body. You barely use your legs in swimming for distances much more than a hundred yards. After that distance the legs are used principally for balance. So if you have severe arthritis of your lower extremities, swimming is a godsend. But if you're trying to build up the strength of your legs, don't count on much of a training effect. To build leg strength, try adding fins.

Swimming with Fins If you suffer from kneecap pain, this is a terrific exercise. Says John Atkins, physical therapist at the Steadman Hawkins Clinic, "As far as really building up the patellar tendon without stressing and forcing the kneecap against the bony prominences of the leg, swimming with fins and a kickboard is just the best thing anyone can do." By adding the extra leverage with the fins, you're not going to be banging your knee around. You instantly start a little more straight-legged and more controlled because you have to control the fins. And by doing that you really develop the hamstrings, the glutes, the upper hamstring attachment. So what you are doing is learning how to control your knees and legs. You can use a very limited range of knee motion and still get a good workout. You can't suddenly load up the knee and damage it like you can with a misstep in running.

Pool Running Once you're in the pool, consider finishing your workout with slow-form running, where you are basically walking across the pool, lifting your knees nice and high. Slow-form running will stretch your low back. You'll be stretching your hamstrings because you are lifting your knee higher than you ever have. In jogging or power walking, you lift your knee only two inches. There's not much range of motion there. But in a pool you can act as though you are an Olympic runner: you can pick up that knee nice and high as if you were sprinting. After two weeks, you'll find yourself moving a little more athletically and naturally picking up your knee a little bit. I once visited the San Francisco 49ers rehab program. Just days after a serious injury, players are in the pool running laps. The ability to do high-speed training without their full body weight is a safe and effective way of getting these players back faster and better.

These aquatic exercises offer a healthy and ultimately safe way to work out. Since the body is virtually weightless in water, trauma to the joints is eliminated. What's more, the increased resistance of water is twelve times as great than that of land-based exercise and can provide for a more effective workout.

Rowing

I love rowing. It allows me to tax every major muscle group in my body. It's rightfully called the "king of aerobic sports" for its amazing ability to tax your heart and lungs to their max. True, many people complain of back and knee pain, but if you have the proper instruction it's a fabulous combination aerobic and weight-training workout. Good technique minimizes the strain. You can get amazing functional range of motion with your knees, bending them to well over 120 degrees. The great advantage here is that you're loading the knee without placing your weight over it. That means you can load it to the maximum amount you feel comfortable with, without fear that a brief stumble will wrench your knee. As in cycling, you do a tremendous amount of work without the strain of a heavy workload during each individual stroke. A high rowing rate or cadence allows you to tax your body and keep the load light. Rowing allows you to get into a full squat position without danger. The best of the rowing trainers is the Concept Two. Try before you buy to see if it works for you.

Elliptical Trainers

The elliptical walker has taken the place of the stair machine for many patients with arthritis. If you have arthritis, consider an elliptical trainer. Still, be careful which one you use. I've found that my kneecaps are burning after using some. It all comes down to the design of the machine. If proper ergonometric principles are used, there's little problem and your joints will feel as they did when you were eighteen. You can also vary the grade and resistance to find a sweet spot for your joints. If you're experiencing pain with a high incline grade, try a lower one. Or try the reverse; a higher grade with a lower load and higher pace. Also, try alternating between walking forward and backward. I've tried several popular brands. Precor doesn't create a lot of motion at the knee joint and doesn't put a lot of load on the joint. If you have really sore kneecaps, you'll find that elliptical trainers can provide glorious relief. I found that some can be used with virtually no knee flexion. Kevin Wilk weighs in: "The elliptical is probably better than the stair climber; most people can tolerate that." Mickey Levinson also advocates them: "I certainly use the elliptical cross-trainer very often. You're getting some of the same muscle activity you'd be getting from running without the impact load, which is a big deal."

StarTrac I've found this elliptical trainer easy on the knees. It allows you to push your leg forward for the beginning of the stride so that your foot actually descends, taking pressure off the knee. The StarTrac has a fluid nonimpact motion and a long stride and simulates the range of motion in the hips, knees, and ankles of jogging or running while minimizing strain on the back.

Again, the elliptical trainer is a little like the StairMaster in that there are ways to cheat on it so you can just ride on the straight leg or what I think of as "riding on your bones." So you have to learn good form.

It's estimated that you can burn up to 720 calories an hour on an elliptical trainer. A recent study of four prominent machines did not show a greater aerobic benefit on any one machine than on the others.

As this book goes to press, there is one amazing new elliptical trainer made by StairMaster—amazing in that the steps actually freely float throughout each step so that you're not riding a rail. This gives you much more freedom in using your joints and in potentially preventing damage to them.

Shoes I asked Mario Lafortune of Nike's Sports Research Lab what to wear. His advice was to wear a lightweight running shoe with *lots* of forefoot padding and very good cushioning. He recommended Nike's Air Pegasus. If you overpronate, you may need either an insert or a different shoe that has better motion control. The Nike Air Kantara and Air Durham incorporate features such as a dual-density midsole, external heel counter, and footbridges to enhance the stability of the foot. Others advise volleyball or court shoes for stair machines.

Scooters

There's no sight on earth more endearing than that of my seven-year-old son scootering in front of me up East Eighty-sixth Street in New York where we live. He throws his right leg in front of his hip as his foot dives for the pavement. He quickly accelerates, ducking and weaving between pedestrians. He makes his Razor fly. Once he said, "Dad, why don't we write a book about scootering?" I told him I'd write about it in my next book. So here goes. They are terrific portable exercise gear. I've taken mine to Chile, much of Africa, Pakistan, and the Middle East. Scooters fold up easily in a suitcase. I use a scooter that has large wheels and a solid base and allows a longer, safer, more comfortable workout. Scootering is a very-low-impact, highly aerobic activity. I seek out hills to increase the workout. Scooters are a dream alternative to walking if your joints hurt while walking. If you're an adult, try the XCooter, a plush adult scooter.

POSSIBLY JOINT-FRIENDLY SPORTS

These sports can be terrific for some and disastrous for others. The difference can be found in fatal flaws you may have and the way your body works. To find if they work for you is often a matter of trial and error.

Stair Machines

Orthopedic surgeons have a love-hate relationship with stair machines. I use them to get into shape for tennis, skiing, surfing, and other sports that require explosive leg strength. However, the stair climber can increase the contact force between the femur and the kneecap. If you have kneecap discomfort due to patellofemoral joint disease when you are on the stair machine, it's not for you, says Dr. Evan Ekman of the Southern Orthopaedic Sports Medicine Center.

I have a stair machine in my study at home and find it a remarkable way to work while I'm working out. I'll read medical journals, research stories on the Web, and read the newspaper. I have found three things that make my knees hurt:

◆ **Foot roll.** If your foot rolls too far to the inside, it pulls your kneecap with it. I fixed my problem by wearing a sports orthotic while using the machine. I also aim at landing squarely on the middle of my foot.

◆ **Sprinting.** Whenever I try to do interval training on the stair machine instead of sticking with a steady pace, I end up with sore kneecaps.

◆ **Letting my knee get too far in front of my foot.**

Patients with mild arthritis can probably use a stair machine safely. Short, choppy steps allow you to get a good workout with a small range of knee motion. Be careful not to bottom out since you'll have to load up your opposite knee.

The middle range of motion seems to be the easiest on the joint, says Kevin Wilk. That means keeping the steps themselves short.

As you get stronger, you can try for a longer step, using pain and discomfort as your guide. If you experience no knee pain, the stair machine is still a magnificent way of building great power and strength. I can train through the fall on the stair machine, then get onto snow in November fully conditioned for skiing—literally as if I'd been skiing all year.

Treadmill

Running The treadmill fundamentally alters the way you walk or run. Scientists call this altering gait mechanics. In the June 2000 issue of *BioMechanics Magazine,* William P. Orien, D.P.M., currently practicing in Bentley Hills, California, wrote that "the growing use of treadmills as an exercise modality, both in health clubs and at home, has paralleled an increase in the number of patients seen with activity-related problems. These symptoms commonly appear as heel, arch, and metatarsal pain, as well as knee and low back problems." Despite the growing number of studies, there are still many unanswered questions regarding the safety of treadmills.

Here's what investigators have found. There is a quickened rate of striding and a decrease in stride length. This requires more steps per mile than running over ground. That means more heel strikes, more push-offs, and more energy expended than when running over ground. Orien concludes, "This may benefit the cardiovascular system, but in anyone with inherent mechanical flaws, the additional repetitious movement may be harmful." The conclusion is simple: if you develop back, knee, ankle, or foot pain, discontinue use of the treadmill until you've seen your doctor! Overall, running on the ground looks to be less traumatic than using a treadmill.

Walking One way around the pounding and altered joint mechanics of running on a treadmill is to walk on it and use the treadmill's incline to increase the intensity of your workout. This maximizes muscle load while minimizing joint impact. Walking on the treadmill uphill at a 7 to 12 percent grade at whatever pace is comfortable gives you the best workout with the least stress to the joints. If you have moderate arthritis of the hip, this could still be too much strain. Trial and error is the most reasonable approach. And don't forget about walking backward as an alternative. A mixed program of running and walking also cuts the demand on your joints. Try a program of four minutes forward to one minute backward. I find this easy on my knees but painful for my hip. For that reason, I walk on a treadmill only as the last alternative. This doesn't mean you shouldn't try treadmill walking if it doesn't cause pain.

Walking

"To say that everyone should walk may be the wrong message," says Dr. Cheryl Riegger-Krugh. Why? The greatest source of wear and tear for many of us can be just plain walking, since that's the activity we do most of. Day in, day out, the tens of thousands of steps we take can wear away our joints. Experts point out that the human joint is designed to endure a hundred years of continuous use without wearing out. It is, but only if the joint stresses created by walking are mechanically perfect.

What goes wrong? "If you're walking incorrectly, you'll just speed up wear-and-tear arthrosis," says Dr. Eric Radin. While many doctors feel that walking is always helpful, Dr. Riegger-Krugh disagrees. "I think if you have a real skeletal misalignment and/or repetitive impulse loading, walking actually could *cause* your arthritis." How? If your gait is mechanically incorrect or you have fatal flaws, abnormal and increased forces can tweak your joints and cause damage.

Risks Versus Benefits The reason many doctors are reluctant to warn patients against walking is that it still has substantial benefits—and they want to be sure that small risks don't prevent patients from accruing major benefits. Dr. Marian Minor correctly points out that "no one has ever proved that walking makes anything worse."

The conclusion I draw from this is that walking is a whole lot better than doing nothing. But given a choice, I do an activity such as biking or in-line skating that puts less stress on the joints. Still, walking can be made much safer for many people by following the steps in this book. Using a well-cushioned walking shoe, getting down to your ideal weight, and improving the way you walk can all decrease the long-term risks of walking.

My Own Experience I shied away from walking for almost a year. After losing eighteen pounds, adding leg strength and flexibility, changing my stride, and buying shock-absorbing shoes, I find I can walk easily without pain. I chose walking as fitness activity of last resort, preferring not to take a chance that I'm still doing silent damage. That's because I already have arthritis in one hip and a rigid foot. Review Chapter 3 to see if there are reasons why walking may not be right for you.

Running

Running? You've got to be crazy! you might say. Running must rip the joints apart! While I might agree with you if you have real biomechanical flaws such as a very rigid foot or are extremely knock-kneed, the fact is that studies do not show that moderate running causes arthritis. If anything, the better the runner, the thicker the cartilage and the better he or she does over the long haul. The smart money says that in running you absorb much of the shock with strong muscles that spare your joints. You are also keeping your muscles elastic, actually creating more shock-absorbing capabilities with the repetitive motion.

Researchers have looked at runners to see how much arthritis they develop. Runners do self-select for their sport. Someone who has a light, flawless frame and a superb, effortless running style may make running a lifetime sport, especially if he or she is free of major injuries. The frequency of osteoarthritis does not differ for runners than for nonrunners or sedentary people, reports Dr. Benno Nigg. Contrast that to a heavy person with a foot that over-pronates and a leg length discrepancy. That person may have pain from the very first run and find it a cumbersome, unwieldy activity. He or she won't stay in the sport for long.

Twenty years ago, I made a decision *not* to run. Why? To be blunt, fear of arthritis. In retrospect I wonder if I wouldn't have maintained more flexibility and had less wear and tear if I'd kept it up. But with a rigid foot and some minor knee injuries, I still think it was a smart move. Some researchers disagree and believe that maintaining motion may help to maintain the bones' normal response to growth. A study backs them up, showing that people who stopped running had more evidence of bone spurs than the people who were still moving.

Not every study gives running a clean bill of health. A University of South Carolina School of Public Health study found that "high levels of physical activity (running 20 or more miles per week) were associated with osteoarthritis among men under age 50." Recreational runners with lesser mileage have not been found to have a higher rate of arthritis. Epidemiological studies of low-impact activity in normal joints, such as recreational jogging, suggest no increase in the risk of self-reported knee-joint pain or X-ray evidence of arthritis. The key phrase is "in normal joints."

A key factor may be undetected old injuries. Recreational runners with a microfracture in the cartilage or a small injury to the bone underlying the cartilage may be predisposed to progressive cartilage wear. In addition, Gabriella Wernicke, M.D., and Richard Panush, M.D., of Saint Barnabas Medical Center noted in the *Bulletin on the Rheumatic Diseases* that running can impact the musculoskeletal system, especially if you have a fatal flaw. They state, "Considering that excessive pronation increases stress on the medial structures of the ankle, shin and knee, and dissipation of the 110 tons of energy by the foot with each mile run, the combination of increased pronation and the large load experienced in the lower extremity increases the risk of overuse injury."

Running Surfaces Different surfaces have different effects on the joints, as follows:

Cinder. This type of surface was the standard track material through the 1970s, when it was replaced with rubberized surfaces. Cinder tracks are preferred for training as they are very forgiving and easy on the joints and muscles, thus also making them very slow when compared with today's surfaces. Cinders are made of ashes mixed with dirt or crushed stone found in reservoirs or rock quarries. Pat Nunan says, "Cinder was one of the best. I mean, they were slow as heck but they were easy on the body." Many cinder tracks have been replaced by polyurethane synthetic athletic surfaces.

Concrete. "The worse surface is concrete, concrete is the least forgiving," says Dr. Nunan.

Asphalt. This is a little better than concrete, depending on how fresh it is.

Brick. Brick is pretty hard, harder than asphalt.

Full-depth, poured-in-place polyurethane synthetic athletic surface. A track such as the one at the Harvard Murr Center Facility is an example of these high-level polyurethane tracks. Some are designed for excellent shock absorption. The best, such as Harvard's running track, are engineered to blunt the impact of running while improving speed.

Grass and dirt. Considered one of the best surfaces, with one caveat: if you have weak muscles or preexisting joint damage, the uneven surface can do further damage to your legs.

The Bottom Line Before you quit running, see if there are any correctable problems such as excess weight or foot problems that are creating a major biomechanical error. Before you take up running, check yourself for the fatal flaws in Chapter 3.

JOINT-UNFRIENDLY SPORTS

These sports load the knee and hip with high impact and large twisting movements.

Tennis

There's no getting around the torque required to play a good game of tennis. If you really enjoy the game and suffer lots of pain, there are several solutions.

Making Tennis More Joint-Friendly One way is to drill with a very good pro so you don't have to do lots of running and readjusting. Just have the pro direct all of the shots directly to you. The other, if you love the game, is to accept that you'll have to do lots of conditioning to play. I'd given up the game, but after six months of yoga, I got back into it pretty much pain free. If you develop a powerful baseline game, you'll remain competitive and spare your joints from added wear and tear.

Skiing

I know a seventy-five-year-old lifetime skiing enthusiast from Montreal. Every morning at 7:30, even at 20 degrees below zero, he's on the quad heading up Mount Mansfield, Vermont's highest peak. Several years ago he was limited to four runs. Why? Knee pain. Skiing had always been a sport with lots of torque or twisting and it had certainly taken its toll on him. That's how you turned the skis. They just *killed* your knees. A friend of mine on the U.S. Ski Team board of directors spends as much time icing his knees after skiing as he does skiing!

He thought his best skiing years were behind him. Now he's back to twelve or more runs a day. What made the difference? The skis.

Making Skiing More Joint-Friendly Shaped skis have made a world of difference. Why? Properly skied, there is virtually no torque at all. By laying the ski over on its side and allowing it to make the turn, there's little torque or twisting movement. I've been able to get back into skiing as a painless activity with shaped skis. It's critical, though, to take carving lessons. Most top skiers believe they do carve, but a close look shows some skidding of the ski, and that means twisting movements of the knee. The key is having the patience to allow the turn to develop and the ski to turn on its own. Good skis and well-groomed terrain make skiing a joint-friendly sport.

Team Sports

A study of former elite-class athletes in Finland found that team-sport athletes had a higher risk of developing knee pain, disability, and arthritis. There's little question that team sports can be the joint-unfriendliest of all. Let's take a look.

Basketball Basketball is tremendously demanding on the joints. Its hard landings, twisting, and shearing can rip up cartilage years before its time. As you age, the loss of elasticity in your muscles and ligaments limits your ability to absorb these forces.

Volleyball As in basketball, the jumping and landing place great stress on the knees. The kneecap in particular "is continually under stress," says Dr. Nancy Major of the Department of Radiology/Department of Surgery Division of Orthopaedics at Duke University.

Football Football players destroy their cartilage much earlier than the regular population, depending on the position they play. "Down lineman, the front line, they have a tendency to wear out their knees more quickly," says Dr. Major. The best protection is having intact knee cartilage, especially the main cushioning pad called the meniscus. It used to be that if you tore your meniscus, your surgeon just took it out. Then doctors discovered the devastating effects of that, which led to very quick arthritis. So now there's a lot of emphasis on sparing as much of the meniscus as possible. Once cartilage is damaged, there is a major increase in the risk of arthritis. If you've played football and injured your knee, choose the joint-friendliest sports you can to minimize wear and tear.

Soccer In Europe, where the sport has long been popular, soccer players develop a degenerative disease in their hips much earlier than the average population. Making images of the joint using magnetic resonance imaging, doctors confirm these changes at these younger ages. This may be the tip of the iceberg. "Unfortunately, in our society we try to be more active and find it important to get our kids involved in these things earlier, but we don't know what the long-term effects are going to be," says Dr. Major.

THE WEEKEND WARRIOR

The last of the true amateur athletes, where no risk is too great for the greater glory of sport. The trouble is this: training for weekend warriors is not as sophisticated or as regular as an elite athlete. Weekend warriors are just not as well prepared. For instance, trained marathon runners have a much thicker cartilage in their knees than someone who just runs occasionally. They stretch appropriately so that they don't have an imbalance of their musculature, which ultimately leads to problems with the knee alignments and kneecap tracking abnormalities. And little wonder: a person who just jogs a few miles a week is not going to invest all the extra time to appropriately balance his or her muscles.

So what are you saying, Dr. Bob, that I have to give up my favorite sports? No! More and more professional athletes are extending their careers. Even baseball players can make it into their late thirties. What I am saying is that if you want to continue to play sports that place large, twisting loads on your joints, you'll have to do a lot more maintenance. You're safer favoring more of the joint-friendly sports for regular training, but for the true weekend warrior being safe is not the goal! Follow the measures in this book, and you'll stand a much better chance of being a weekend warrior and still not limping to work on Monday.

14

Conclusion

A senior NBC correspondent had just come back from a long, hard two months in Afghanistan. "Foreign correspondent? That's a young man's game," he told me outside his office in a weary way. It *is* a young man's game, I thought. You need boundless energy, strong, supple muscles, and the joints of a teenager. I didn't have the heart to tell him I'd been offered the dream assignment of a lifetime—special foreign correspondent out in the most rugged and dangerous parts of the world: the hottest hot spots, from Afghanistan and Somalia to the wilds of Ethiopia, Yemen, the Himalayas and Sudan. With the elite of America's army special forces, with the navy chasing smugglers in Iraqi territorial waters, with the air force in the skies over Afghanistan. A year ago I would have had to turn the assignment down. With a bum hip, a distinct limp, and little mobility in most of my joints, I would have been a liability at best. I recalled the painful climb up the volcano on Hokkaido in 1999. Now I'm as good as I've ever been. I am playing the young man's game and with relish. On the road, I put in regular twenty-two-hour days and hiked dozens of miles in nearly impassable mountainous terrain. I thank the steps in this book for getting me there. I race through airports or along rocky riverbeds in my air-soled running shoes. Each night before bed, I restore my joints with yoga. Each morning I take my supplements faithfully to help rebuild my cartilage. I've put the spring back in my step with plyometrics. Beating wear and tear has made a world of difference for me, making the impossible possible—and I'm sure it will for you as well.

APPENDIX: JOINT NUTRITION

I'm often a target of the self-appointed food police. "Gee, isn't that a Ring Ding?" my thirteen-year-old son will accuse me. Complete strangers will come up to me in disbelief if I'm caught at a fast-food restaurant with my kids and say, "Gee, Dr. Bob, you eat hamburgers?" There's no escaping it. I'm aware of the ever-watchful eye of the nutritionally correct public, so I do try my best to eat right. In the paneled elegance of the Los Angeles Sports Club, two very attractive sisters once accosted me in a friendly way. "Gee, that looks *really* healthy," said one about my edamame appetizer, tomato juice cocktail, and sea bass with sweet potatoes main course. The other joined in: "So is this a heart-healthy diet?" "Nope," I admitted. "Cancer prevention?" asked the other. Wrong again. Of course, it would have served either purpose, but this was a *joint-healthy* diet, really a new concept for even the most nutritionally aware.

The conventional wisdom: Joint nutrition is a waste of time and money.

The real deal: Nutrients are the font of life for your joints.

We're all eager to find supplements that may improve our joints. We've looked at the most powerful in Chapters 6 and 7. There are other nutrients that may be of some benefit. The evidence for most of these is preliminary and thin, which is why you'll find them here in the appendix. However, the case for taking an adequate amount of these common vitamins for your general health is strong. Although many of these supplements claim to treat osteoarthritis, the Arthritis Foundation has reviewed each product along with its scientific rationale and given insight into those supplements that look most promising. The AF experts singled out a few of these supplements as "ones worth considering." However, they state, "Before trying any of them, talk to your doctor about which would be right for you. Those that are said to be worth considering by the arthritis association are marked (AF). The foundation has had an expert panel review all of the claims against the actual scientific evidence. The Arthritis Foundation recommends trying one new supplement at a time and keeping a record of its effects, noting the brand and dose. After three months on any supplement, be sure to have a medical evaluation to check for side effects. Don't overdose. More is not better. Be sure your doctor is aware of every supplement that you are taking. Many interact with medications and some could interfere if you are having surgery. You'll note some interfere with your blood clotting system. In particular, researchers are quite concerned about the megadosing of antioxidants. Very preliminary studies hint that megadoses of beta-carotene or vitamin C might help fuel tumor growth.

CARTILAGE REPAIR

Antioxidants: Vitamins C, D, and E

Antioxidants may slow oxidative damage to cartilage, so increasing your antioxidant intake may have a positive effect. A study in *Arthritis and Rheumatism* examining the association of dietary intake of antioxidants with the incidence and progression of knee arthritis as measured on X rays, has shown "a threefold reduction in progressive disease in people with higher intake of vitamin C." Dr. Timothy McAlindon says, "Preliminary results from several studies appear particularly strong for vitamin D, and to a lesser extent for vitamin C and vitamin E." Howeyer, vitamin C won't prevent arthritis.

Dosage: *Vitamin C*—Usual dose is 100 milligrams to 1,000 milligrams per day. You may want to stick with a lower dosage unless your doctor okays the higher amount. *Vitamin D*—Usual dosage is 400 IU to 800 IU per day. See below. *Vitamin E*—Usual dosage was 400 IU to 600 IU per day. See below.

RETARDATION OF DISEASE PROGRESSION

Vitamins C, D, and E

Too low an intake of these vitamins is associated with the progression of knee and hip arthritis. Take vitamin D as an example.

Vitamin D (AF)

Researchers found a threefold higher risk of progression of arthritis in participants who had low to medium intakes of vitamin D. Another study found a similar association between low serum vitamin D levels and progression of arthritis of the hip. The entire body surface of our ancestors was exposed to the sun almost daily. Today we cover all but 5 percent of our skin, except in the summer. The further north you live, the less exposure you get to natural sunlight.

There are two ways to make up the difference. Get outside for ten to fifteen minutes a day. Sunblocks *do* block vitamin D absorption. Take a multivitamin containing vitamin D. You don't want to take excess amounts of vitamin D, so the multivitamin really is all you need—and all that's approved by the FDA. A good multivitamin also contains as much vitamins C and E, and beta-carotene as are needed for a good joint nutrition program. Good sources of vitamin D include milk (which contains about 100 IU per cup), fatty fish, fish liver oils, and egg yolks.

Dosage: 400 to 800 IU per day.

Methyl-Sulfonyl-Methane (MSM)

Methyl-sulfonyl-methane is being promoted as a way to help rebuild damaged joint cartilage. MSM is called the natural partner to the glucosamine molecule. Why? Chondroitin is the main component in joint cartilage. MSM and glucosamine are the basic molecules needed for the synthesis of chondroitin.

Be aware that some people may develop allergic responses to MSM. Also, to date, the evidence is thin that MSM is helpful. There are no human studies showing effectiveness. The Arthritis Foundation makes a special point of *not* recommending MSM.

A new abstract presented at the American College of Rheumatology's 65th Annual Scientific Meeting in 2001 did state that drugs such as acetaminophen could enhance the urinary loss of sulfur. For those individuals losing sulfur, enhancing sulfur intake might prove useful. Sulfur is necessary for the normal repair and upkeep of cartilage.

Marc Hochberg adds, "I have not heard any data for the MSM supplement. I certainly wouldn't recommend it."

Judith Horstman, author of *The Arthritis Foundation's Guide to Alternative Therapies,* adds this purchasing advice:

◆ Buy MSM only from an established company that you can be sure will stand by its products—and be wary of companies making "miracle" and other hyped claims.

◆ Start with a low dosage of 500 milligrams or less twice a day and gradually increase the amount until you notice some effect. Most sources suggest 1,000 milligrams (1 gram) twice a day. MSM is most often taken in capsules or dissolved in a liquid.

◆ Be patient. But if you don't see any difference after two months, you may never—and it may not be worth continuing to expose yourself to unknown risks.

◆ Tell your doctor if you get diarrhea, stomach upset, or mild cramps; these side effects are common, especially at higher doses. Lowering the dosage may stop these symptoms.

Side effects: Nausea, diarrhea, headache, stomach upset, mild cramps. Lowering the dose may decrease the side effects.

ConsumerLab.com has also done testing on MSM products.

GENERAL JOINT NUTRIENTS

Niacin (Vitamin B3)

The Arthritis Foundation notes that vitamin B3 can interfere with diabetes drugs, so diabetics should monitor their blood glucose levels carefully. Food sources include lean meat, fish, peanuts, brewer's yeast, and soy.

Niacin is taken for various arthritis symptoms including pain and stiffness. Study shows NSAID dosage could be reduced by 13 percent by taking B3.

Dosage: 10 to 25 milligrams per day.

Vitamin E (AF)

The Arthritis Foundation says that vitamin E is a heart-healthy vitamin and worth considering. Vitamin E, in one study, beat NSAIDs for pain relief. Vitamin E comes in different forms, natural and synthetic. Ask for the natural alpha-tocopherol form.

Recently, one group from Australia found that vitamin E provided no more benefit than placebo in relieving pain. However, the role of vitamin E in preventing osteoarthritis progression is still under investigation. It is possible that vitamin E might stop the loss of joint cartilage and therefore would be protective. The Australia group is now analyzing the data to answer this question.

Dosage: 400 to 600 IU per day.

Manganese

Manganese has been combined with glucosamine and chondroitin. The combination product relieves osteoarthritic pain. It's not known what the effect of manganese is on its own. Don't take more than 11 milligrams a day, says the Arthritis Foundation. High doses might lead to manganese accumulation and symptoms similar to those of Parkinson's disease, including psychosis. People with chronic liver disease should use it cautiously.

The Arthritis Foundation states that a glucosamine-chondroitin-manganese combination has been shown effective for osteoarthritis pain but it's not known if manganese contributes to these results!

Dosage: Adequate intake is 2.3 milligrams per day. More than 11 milligrams a day can be toxic.

Selenium

The Arthritis Foundation says it may be helpful for rheumatoid arthritis (one study showed fewer tender joints, but the subjects were also taking fish oil), but there are no human studies indicating it may be helpful for wear-and-tear arthritis.

Selenium may also help to protect against prostate cancer.

Dosage: 50 to 200 micrograms per day.

Omega-3 Fatty Acids (AF)

Human studies have shown that fish oil can reduce the pain and inflammation of rheumatoid arthritis. What effect it may have on wear-and-tear arthritis is not known. However, omega-3 fatty acids are part of a healthy diet and are a heart-healthy fat. Omega-3 fatty acids are found naturally in oily fish.

Omega-3 fats are available as supplements. To avoid heavy metals, you should buy only supplements that are molecularly distilled. Omega-3 700, made by Solgar, is one such product. I take two capsules a day.

Supplements should be taken with meals. Since these oils do have an effect on blood clotting, review their use with your doctor if you take blood thinners or NSAIDs. A recent report by ConsumerLab.com showed no increased heavy metals in the products tested. See www.consumerlab.com for other specific brand names.

Side effects: Increase the effect of blood thinners and may cause belching, bad breath, heartburn, and nosebleeds. Causes nausea and diarrhea at high doses.

Dosage: Usual dosage is 12 grams.

Green Tea

The claim made for green tea is that it can relieve pain and inflammation. There are no studies showing its effectiveness in humans.

Nonetheless, green tea is chock-full of antioxidants and is being investigated in several clinical trials as an agent to prevent cancer. I take it as a powder each morning, mixed with water.

Side effects: Allergic reactions, upset stomach, constipation.

Bromelain

Bromelain is a potent anti-inflammatory agent that is found in fresh pineapple juice. The claim is that bromelain eases the inflammation of wear-and-tear arthritis. The Arthritis Foundation reports that a product combining bromelain with trypsin and rutin relieved the pain of osteoarthritics as well as NSAIDs did. The Arthritis Foundation says there is one promising animal study for arthritis but no scientific evidence that bromelain alone is effective in humans. It is likely safe. Be wary if you are taking blood-thinning drugs.

Side effects: In higher doses can cause upset stomach or cramps. Avoid if you are allergic to pineapple. Can increase the effect of blood-thinning drugs.

Cetyl Myristoleate (CMO)

The claim is that CMO relieves the symptoms of wear-and-tear arthritis. The Arthritis Foundation says there are no human studies to back up the claim. There is no set dosage. Promoters cite a study showing a 72 percent improvement in "the arthritic condition." When it is taken three times a day for two to four weeks once a year, promoters of CMO say, people gain relief from arthritic symptoms. Technically, CMO is an oil derived from a bovine source of myristoleic fatty acid. It is also found in butter, fish, and whale oils. Its risks are unknown at present.

Side effects: Unknown.

Warning: To avoid irreversible joint damage, do not stop taking prescription medication without talking to your doctor first.

Magnesium

Calcium crystals in the joints can amplify their degradation and eventual destruction. Oral magnesium is reported to lessen symptoms in arthritis where crystal deposition is a problem.

The Arthritis Foundation says a placebo-controlled study of a magnesium and malic acid combination product found that it eased pain and boosted energy in twenty-four women with fibromyalgia.

Chronic fatigue symptoms are connected to low magnesium levels, and supplements have been shown to improve these symptoms.

Side effects: Magnesium can interact with blood pressure medication; may cause loose stools, nausea, vomiting, diarrhea, stomach irritation. Don't use if you have kidney problems because it can cause kidney failure.

Avocado and Soy Oils

These are not mentioned in the Arthritis Foundation guide.

This treatment for osteoarthritis is made from extracts of avocado and soybean. The technical term is avocado/soybean unsaponifiables or ASU. In animals taking these oils, the thickness and quality of cartilage were improved.

A study in humans showed that patients could take fewer NSAIDs if they took ASU. The treatment was more effective in patients with hip arthritis.

In summary, the Arthritis Foundation says that these are supplements worth discussing with your physician for wear-and-tear arthritis.

I'm the first to admit that long lists like the one above make me see red. There are a dozen items most with little real proof they work, leaving you with the feeling that you should do something but without much motivation to act. I take a simple approach: I make sure I get all of the antioxidants listed in high-powered fruits and vegetables. If I'm somewhere where those are not available, I take a multivitamin. I do take fish oil for its heart-healthy effects.

Real Antioxidants from Real Foods (AF)

Many of us just say "ugh" when it comes to even thinking about eating enough fruits and vegetables. Just think of the guilt. We're supposed to eat *nine* servings a day. Most of us are lucky to get one or two. Our kids' top vegetable is the French fry! I've found two easy ways to get antioxidants from real foods. First, eat fruits and vegetables that are richest in antioxidants. You'll find, for example, that one sweet potato is the equivalent of five lesser vegetables. Or look at fruits; cantaloupe and strawberries put many lesser fruits to shame. That being said, the very *easiest* way to get your veggies in one fell swoop is with a blender. Now, before you think, Dr. Bob has started doing late-night cable TV ads, hear me out! The blender I use is the Vitamixer, which allows you to put whole fruits or vegetables into the mixer. Its lawn mower–like power allows you to rip through even the toughest fruits and vegetables. I use tomato juice as a base and then dump in a half dozen different veggies.

GLOSSARY

SOURCES OF DEFINITIONS:

AAOS: American Academy of Orthopaedic Surgeons
AAPM: American Academy of Pain Management (or Medicine)
APMA: American Podiatric Medical Association
NIAMS: National Institute of Arthritis and Musculoskeletal and Skin Diseases
NIH: National Institutes of Health

Analgesic: A medication or treatment that relieves pain.

Anterior cruciate ligament (ACL): In the center of the knee; limits rotation and the forward movement of the tibia. (NIAMS)

Anterior superior iliac spines: The iliac spines are the small bony protuberances at the front of your pelvis. "Anterior" refers to the front of the body and "superior" refers to the top of the body, closer to the head.

Arthritis: Joint problems stemming primarily from metabolic or inflammatory causes.

Arthroscopy: "A procedure performed with an arthroscope (a small, flexible tube that transmits the image of the inside of a joint to a video monitor). Arthroscopy is used for diagnosis as well as treatment of some types of joint injury." (NIAMS)

Arthrosis: Joint problems initially from mechanical abnormalities followed by inflammation, as defined by Dr. Eric Radin.

Blount's disease: A growth disorder of the tibia (the bone at the front of the lower leg, sometimes called the shinbone) that causes the lower leg to angle inward, resembling a bowleg. Blount's disease occurs primarily in young children but can occur during adolescence. The cause is unknown. (NIH)

Bunion: A protrusion of the big toe joint, also known as the metatarsophalangeal joint. Misaligned big toe joints can become swollen and tender, causing the first joint of the big toe to slant outward, and the second joint to angle toward the other toes. Bunions tend to be hereditary, but can be aggravated by shoes that are too narrow in the forefoot and toe.

Bursitis: A condition involving inflammation of the bursae, which are small sacs located between bone and other moving structures such as muscle and tendons.

Cartilage: "A resilient tissue that covers and cushions the ends of the bones and absorbs shock." (NIAMS)

Chondroitin: Chondroitin sulfate is sold as a dietary or nutritional supplement and is a substance that is found naturally in the body. Chondroitin sulfate is part of a large protein molecule (proteoglycan) that gives cartilage elasticity. The supplement comes from cattle trachea (windpipes) or shark cartilage.

Chondromalacia (KON-dro-mah-LAY-she-ah): Also called chondromalaciapatellae; refers to softening of the articular cartilage of the kneecap. This disorder occurs most often in young adults and can be caused by injury, overuse, parts out of alignment, or muscle weakness. Instead of gliding smoothly across the lower end of the thighbone, the kneecap rubs against it, thereby roughening the cartilage underneath the kneecap. (NIAMS)

Collagen: The main structural protein of skin, bones, tendons, cartilage, and connective tissue. (NIAMS)

Collateral ligaments: The collateral ligaments are located at the inner and outer sides of the knee joint. The medial collateral ligament (MCL) connects the thighbone to the shinbone and provides stability to the inner side of the knee. The lateral collateral ligament (LCL) connects the thighbone to the other bone in the lower portion of your leg (fibula) and stabilizes the outer side. (AAOS)

Connective tissue: "The supporting framework of the body and its internal organs." (NIAMS)

Cytokines: Small molecular-weight proteins that mediate communications between cells.

Debridement (arthroscopy): This process consists of washing all debris and loose fragments out of a joint. The loose fragments of cartilage are removed and the knee is washed with a saline (salt) solution.

Developmental hip dysplasia: An abnormal formation of the hip joint in which the ball at the top of the thighbone (femoral head) is not stable in the socket (acetabulum). Also, the ligaments of the hip joint may be loose and stretched.

Femoral groove: The thighbone (femur) has a V-shaped notch (femoral groove or sulcus) at one end to accommodate the moving kneecap. In a normal knee, the kneecap fits nicely in the groove. But if the groove is uneven or too shallow, the kneecap can slide off, resulting in a partial or complete dislocation. A sharp blow to the kneecap, as in a fall, can also pop the kneecap out of place. (AAOS)

Fibroblast: A type of cell found underneath the skin surface. Fibroblasts serve as part of the support structure for tissues and organs.

Genu valgum: An outward deviation of the legs at the knee. It is an acquired deformity. It can be unilateral or bilateral.

Genu varum: A deformity wherein there is lateral bowing of the legs at the knee. Such a bowing at the tibia is called *tibia varum.*

Glucosamine: Glucosamine is sold as a dietary or nutritional supplement and is a substance that is found naturally in the body. It is a form of amino sugar that is believed to play a role in cartilage formation and repair. It is made from the chitin in the shells of crab, lobster, and shrimp.

Hammertoes: Sometimes called clawtoes. A condition usually stemming from muscle imbalance, in which the toes become crooked and bent and start to buckle under, causing the joints to protrude. It occurs most frequently with the second toe, often when a bunion slants the big toe toward and under it, but any of the other three smaller toes can be affected.

Iliotibial band syndrome: An overuse condition in which inflammation results when a band of a tendon rubs over the outer bone (lateral condyle) of the knee. Although iliotibial band syndrome may be caused by direct injury to the knee, it is most often caused by the stress of long-term overuse, such as sometimes occurs in sports training. (NIAMS)

Inflammation: "A typical reaction of tissue to injury or disease. It is marked by four signs: swelling, redness, heat, and pain." (NIAMS)

Joint: "The place where two or more bones are joined. Most joints are composed of cartilage, joint space, fibrous capsule, synovium, and ligaments." (NIAMS)

Joint space: "The area enclosed within the fibrous capsule and synovium." (NIAMS)

Lateral ankle sprain: A sprain of the structures on the outside of the ankle.

Lateral malleolus: The outer bony projection of the small outer bone in the foreleg called the fibula.

Legg-Calvé-Perthes disease: A condition in children in which the top of the thighbone (femoral head) dies from lack of blood supply, becomes brittle, and may collapse, leading to deformity and arthritis. (AAOS)

Magnetic resonance imaging (MRI): "A diagnostic technique that provides high-quality cross-sectional images of a structure of the body without X rays or other radiation." (NIAMS)

Malalignment: The alignment of the hip, knee, and ankle influences how the knee reacts to loads. A knee that is turned inward or outward is susceptible to added stress. When it is not normally positioned, it is malaligned.

Malleolus: A rounded projection from a bone.

Medial knee pain: Pain on the inside of the knee.

Medial malleolus: The inner bony projection of the ankle.

Meniscal tear: A meniscal tear is characterized by a traumatic or degenerative tear of the medial or lateral meniscus. Meniscal tears may occur in isolation or in association with a ligament injury or fracture. (AAOS)

Meniscus: Separating the bones of the knee are pads of connective tissue. One pad is called a meniscus (muh-NISS-kus). The plural is menisci (muh-NISS-sky). The menisci are divided into two crescent-shaped discs positioned between the tibia and femur on the outer and inner sides of each knee (the medial and the lateral menisci). The two menisci in each knee act as shock absorbers, cushioning the lower part of the leg from the weight of the rest of the body as well as enhancing stability. (NIAMS)

Metatarsal stress fracture: A break in a bone caused by repetitive stress. It may occur in any bone but is quite common in the metatarsal bones of the foot (metatarsal bones are similar to the knuckles in your hand).

Microklutziness: Micro-incoordination of neuromuscular control not visible to the naked eye, as defined by Dr. Eric Radin.

Neuroma: An enlarged benign growth on a nerve, most commonly between the third and fourth toes. It is caused by tissue rubbing against and irritating the nerves. Pressure from ill-fitting shoes or abnormal bone structure can create the condition as well. (APMA)

Nonsteroidal anti-inflammatory drugs (NSAIDs): A group of medications, including aspirin, ibuprofen, and related drugs, used to reduce inflammation that causes joint pain, stiffness, and swelling. (NIAMS)

Osteoarthritis: "Also known as degenerative joint disease. Osteoarthritis primarily affects cartilage, which is the tissue that cushions the ends of bones within the joint. Osteoarthritis occurs when cartilage begins to fray, wear, and decay. In extreme cases, the cartilage may wear away entirely, leaving a bone-on-bone joint." (NIAMS)

Osteonecrosis: Osteonecrosis of the hip is a disabling condition that can lead to the hip joint collapsing. The condition may start with few signs or warnings. If one has osteonecrosis of the hip, the blood vessels gradually cut off nourishment to the top of the thighbone (femur) where it fits in the hip socket. Without blood, the head of the femur dies and collapses. This can make it painful to move the hip, and a person suffering from it may develop arthritis and a limp. Cartilage in the hip socket may also break down. The same problems generally develop in the other hip. (AAOS)

Patellofemoral (kneecap) pain syndrome: A group of conditions that characterize pain beneath or surrounding the patella resulting from physical or biochemical changes. Patellofemoral pain is the most common source of knee pain. Although patellofemoral pain is often mislabeled as chondromalacia, it is important to distinguish it from chondromalacia, which is actual damage to the patellar cartilage. Sources of pain include patella malalignment, osteoarthritis, osteochondral fractures, synovial plica, bursitis, tendonitis, and patella instability.

Plantar fasciitis: Plantar fasciitis (heel pain) is commonly traced to an inflammation on the bottom of the foot. (AAPM)

Repetitive impulse loading (RIL): Hard-and-fast joint loading with inadequate shock absorption, as defined by Dr. Cheryl Riegger-Krugh.

Rheumatoid arthritis: "An inflammatory disease of the synovium, or lining of the joint, that results in pain, stiffness, swelling, deformity, and loss of function in the joints." (NIAMS)

Shinsplits: Microtears in or inflammation of the anterior leg muscles. Pain on either side of the leg bone, caused by muscle or tendon inflammation. It is commonly related to excessive foot pronation (collapsing arch) but may be related to a muscle imbalance between opposing muscle groups in the leg. (APMA)

Slipped capital femoral epiphysis: The most common hip disorder among young teenagers. SCFE occurs when the cartilage plate (epiphysis) at the top of the child's thighbone (femur) slips out of place. In a growing child, the plate is what controls which way the top of the thigh-bone grows. It's also a pivotal part of the hip's ball-and-socket joint, so slippage of the epiphysis may severely deform the child. (AAOS)

Tibial tuberosity: The roughened protuberance on the shin bone (tibia) just below the knee. It attaches to the patellar ligament, which serves as the insertion of the quadriceps femoris tendon.

SELECTED BIOGRAPHIES

The American Academy of Podiatric Sports Medicine (AAPSM) was founded in San Francisco in 1970 by a group of podiatric sports physicians who had the insight to realize the need for a podiatric sports medicine association devoted to the treatment of athletic injuries. Today the AAPSM has more than eight hundred members. It is the second-largest affiliate organization of the American Podiatric Medical Association. With the emerging awareness of a fitness-oriented society, sports podiatry helped to shift the emphasis of sports medicine away from its purely surgical past. The concepts of prevention and biomechanics helped to change the focus of the modern practice of sports medicine. Web site: www.aapsm.org

The American College of Sports Medicine (ACSM) is an association of people and professions sharing the commitment to explore the use of medicine and exercise to make life healthier for all Americans. ACSM's mission is to promote and integrate scientific research, education, and practical applications of sports medicine and exercise science to maintain and enhance physical performance, fitness, health, and quality of life. Web site: www.acsm.org

The Arthritis Foundation is the only national not-for-profit organization that supports the more than one hundred types of arthritis and related conditions with advocacy, programs, services, and research. The mission of the Arthritis Foundation is to improve lives through leadership in the prevention, control, and cure of arthritis and related diseases. Web site: www.arthritis.org

John Atkins is a certified athletic trainer with a master's degree in sports medicine and physical education. He has worked with the U.S. ski team over the past twenty years as director of conditioning, head trainer, and currently team-building consultant. Atkins is codirector of the Steadman Hawkins Clinic in Vail, Colorado.

Kenneth Brandt, M.D., is one of the leading OA experts in the nation. He is the director of the Indiana University Multipurpose Arthritis Center as well as the head of the Rheumatology Division and Musculoskeletal Diseases Center.

Gary Brazina, M.D., also known as "The Jock Doc," is a Los Angeles–based board-certified orthopedic surgeon who specializes in arthroscopic surgery and sports medicine. He is a fellow of the American Academy of Orthopaedic Surgeons and the American College of Surgeons. Dr. Brazina has more than twenty years of surgical experience and has treated some of the United States' top athletes.

Yogiraj Bikram Choudhury is the founder of the Yoga College of India. Born in Calcutta in 1946, Bikram began yoga at the age of four with Bishnu Ghosh, brother of Paramahansa Yogananda. Bikram practiced yoga four to six hours a day with six thousand other students at Ghosh's College of Physical Education in Calcutta, and at the age of thirteen, he won the National India Yoga Contest. He was undefeated for three years. Bikram was asked by Ghosh to start several yoga schools in India. There Bikram came into his own. The schools were so successful that at Ghosh's request Bikram traveled to Japan and opened two more. He has since taken his curative methods of yoga therapy around the world.

Frank A. Cordasco, M.D., is an orthopedic surgeon in the Sports Medicine and Shoulder Service at the Hospital for Special Surgery, New York City, and an associate professor of orthopedic surgery at the Weill Medical College of Cornell University, New York City. He has been in practice since 1990, specializing in surgery for sports-related injuries of the knee and shoulder.

Cooper Institute, a nonprofit research and education center, conducts research in epidemiology, exercise physiology, behavior change, hypertension, children's health, obesity, nutrition, aging, and other health issues. Papers from the Cooper Institute are among the most frequently cited references in the scientific literature on topics related to physical fitness, physical activity, and health. Research conducted at the institute has influenced major national public policy initiatives from the American Heart Association, the American College of Sports Medicine, and the Centers for Disease Control and Prevention. The Cooper Institute has more than six hundred articles and manuscripts in peer-reviewed journals and lay publications, with approximately fifty publications per year in each of the last five years. Web site: www.cooperinst.org

Howard J. Dananberg, D.P.M., is a podiatrist in Bedford, New Hampshire. He is renowned for his research and treatment protocols on walking style and chronic postural pain and serves as a contributing editor to the *Journal of the American Podiatric Medical Association*.

Colonel Gail Deyle, M.P.T., is the chief of physical therapy at Brooke Army Medical Center at Fort Sam Houston in San Antonio, Texas, and a senior faculty member at the U.S. Army–Baylor University Doctor of Science Program in Orthopaedic Physical Therapy. Colonel Deyle has a B.S. degree in biology from the University of Nebraska at Kearney, a master of physical therapy degree from Baylor University, and a doctor of physical therapy degree from Creighton University.

Natalie D. Eddington, Ph.D., is an associate professor of pharmaceutics and the director of the Pharmacokinetics-Biopharmaceutics Laboratory in the School of Pharmacy at the University of Maryland, Baltimore. She served as an assistant director of clinical drug development at Pfizer Pharmaceuticals and later joined the faculty of the University of Maryland. Her research interests include examining factors that influence drug delivery and pharmacokinetics of drugs across biological membranes using in vitro cell culture, animal models, and healthy volunteers so as to elucidate structure-pharmacokinetic and pharmacodynamic relationships. Dr. Eddington also studies the pharmacokinetic issues of dietary supplements and botanical agents in terms of their evaluation and possible drug interactions.

Evan F. Ekman, M.D., is the director of the Southern Orthopaedic Sports Medicine Center in Columbia, South Carolina. Dr. Ekman is a fellow of the American Academy of Orthopaedic Surgeons. He is a recipient of the John Joyce Award from the International Society of Arthroscopy, Knee Surgery and Orthopaedic Sports Medicine as well as the Allen Lacy Endowment from the Southern Orthopaedic Association.

William Evans, M.D., is a professor of geriatrics, physiology, and nutrition and the director of the Nutrition, Metabolism and Exercise Laboratory at the University of Arkansas for Medical Sciences. He has authored more than 160 scientific publications as well as *AstroFit,* published by Simon & Schuster in spring 2002.

Joseph H. Feinberg, M.D., is a physiatrist at the Hospital for Special Surgery in New York City. Dr. Feinberg also holds a master's degree in biochemistry. He has served as the team physician of St. Peter's College in Jersey City, New Jersey, since 1992 and has served as the team physician for Seton Hall University (1995–1997), the professional soccer team the Jersey Dragons (1994–1996), and Jersey City State College (1995–1999). Dr. Feinberg has completed fellowships in orthopedic pathology and orthopedic biomechanics. His superspecialties include peripheral nerve disorders, electrodiagnostic testing, and spine- and sports-related conditions. Dr. Feinberg's area of research interest is muscle fatigue.

Sharon Feldmann, M.S., PT, OCS, has worked at the Rehabilitation Institute of Chicago since 1989, starting out as a staff physical therapist. She is currently the clinical manager of the Arthritis Center. Her publications include the chapter "Exercise for the Person with Rheumatoid Arthritis," in R. W. Chang, ed., *Rehabilitation of Persons with Rheumatoid Arthritis*. In addition, she has presented papers at the Rehabilitation Institute of Chicago's annual course, "Excellence in Joint Replacement," for five years. She has also facilitated many community-based programs and seminars, including exercise courses and patient education classes.

David Felson, M.D., M.P.H., is a rheumatologist and clinical epidemiologist who is an expert in osteoarthritis epidemiology and treatment. Dr. Felson is one of the most prominent arthritis researchers in the world. He founded and leads the Framingham Osteoarthritis Study, a major study of risk factors for osteoarthritis. He is professor of medicine and public health at Boston University School of Medicine and chair of the Clinical Epidemiology Research and Training Unit at Boston Medical Center in Boston.

Marian Garfinkel, M.D., is a specialist in the prevention of repetitive strain injuries. She is a faculty lecturer at MCP Hahnemann University and researcher at the University of Pennsylvania Medical School. Dr. Garfinkel contributes to various newsletters, periodicals, and journals in the United States and abroad. Her study on carpal tunnel syndrome was published in the *Journal of the American Medical Association*. She is the director of the B. K. S. Iyengar Yoga Studio of Philadelphia and a senior Iyengar yoga teacher, assessor, and teacher trainer. She has traveled to India annually since 1974 to study with B. K. S. Iyengar and his children, Geeta and Prashant.

Allan Gelber, M.D., M.P.H., Ph.D., is an assistant professor of medicine in the Division of Rheumatology at Johns Hopkins University School of Medicine in Baltimore, Maryland. His research interests include the incidence and risk factors for osteoarthritis; the effect of a home-based exercise intervention for knee osteoarthritis in an inner-city

African-American community located in Baltimore, Maryland; and the prevalence of osteoarthritis and Raynaud's phenomenon in the African-American community.

James E. Graves, Ph.D., is the associate dean for graduate studies, budget, and research as well as a professor of exercise science at Syracuse University. Dr. Graves is a prolific author in the field of exercise science. He is cofounder of the Center for Exercise Science at the University of Florida and founder of the Musculoskeletal Laboratory at Syracuse University. His most recent publication is *Resistance Training for Health and Rehabilitation*, published by Human Kinetics.

Topper Hagerman, Ph.D., sports physiologist, has spent the last twenty-five years working in the sports medicine field, focusing on fitness, training programs, injury prevention, and health and wellness research. He is currently codirector of the Steadman Hawkins Clinic in Vail, Colorado.

Howard J. Hillstrom, Ph.D., received a B.S. in electrical engineering from Worcester Polytechnic Institute (WPI) in 1978, an M.S. in biomedical engineering from WPI in 1980, and a Ph.D. from Drexel University in 1989. Currently Dr. Hillstrom directs the Gait Study Center at the Temple University School of Podiatric Medicine in Philadelphia, Pennsylvania. His research investigates the biomechanical relationship between lower-extremity structure and function with special attention to the patient with rheumatic disease.

Marc C. Hochberg, M.D., M.P.H., is a leading arthritis researcher at the University of Maryland School of Medicine in Baltimore, Maryland. Since 1995 he has been the head of the Division of Rheumatology and Clinical Immunology in the Department of Medicine and since 1991 has been a professor of medicine and epidemiology and preventive medicine at the University of Maryland School of Medicine. Dr. Hochberg has received numerous awards and has held appointments in several nationally and internationally acclaimed medical societies. He is a founding fellow of the American College of Rheumatology and a fellow of the American College of Physicians. He received the Clinical Research Award from the Osteoarthritis Research Society International in 1999. In addition, he is on the editorial boards of several journals, including *Rheumatology, Annals of the Rheumatic Diseases, The Journal of Rheumatology, Clinical and Experimental Rheumatology*, and *Osteoarthritis and Cartilage*.

Kenneth Holt, Ph.D., PT, is associate professor and director of the Barreca Motion Analysis Laboratory at Boston University. He studies locomotion in children with cerebral palsy and Down's syndrome, individuals with structural abnormalities of the lower extremity, and the elderly. He also runs a physical therapy practice specializing in biomechanical analysis and orthotic therapy for sufferers of chronic musculoskeletal injury.

Gary R. Hunter, Ph.D., earned his doctorate from Michigan State University and is professor and director of exercise physiology at the University of Alabama at Birmingham. He has published more than 150 research papers concerning metabolism, high-intensity training, and body composition.

Michael Hurley, Ph.D., M.C.S.P., is a physical therapist and a reader in physiotherapy at King's College, London, and head of the Rehabilitation Research Unit, Dulwich Hospital, London. His research interests are muscle dysfunction in patients with traumatic and degenerative joint problems, with a special interest in knee osteoarthritis. The main aim of this research is to develop simple rehabilitation regimes for these common conditions that patients can do in order to self-manage their conditions, thereby maintaining their independence. Funded by the Arthritis Research Campaign, he is running a large clinical trial investigating the clinical and cost effectiveness of rehabilitation of patients with chronic knee pain.

Casey Kerrigan, M.D., is professor and chairman of physical medicine and rehabilitation at the University of Virginia in Charlottesville. Dr. Kerrigan received her medical degree from Harvard Medical School and performed her residency at the University of California at Los Angeles. She has authored numerous scientific investigations on the biomechanics and physiology of human walking, including studies on the effect of women's shoe wear on knee joint torques that may be relevant to the development of knee joint osteoarthritis.

John Klippel, M.D., is the medical director of the Arthritis Foundation. He is also the former clinical director of the National Institute of Arthritis and Musculoskeletal and Skin Diseases (NIAMS), a part of the National Institutes of Health (NIH). Dr. Klippel has more than twenty-five years of experience in rheumatology and biomedical research related to arthritis and has authored numerous scientific and clinical publications.

William Kraemer, Ph.D., is currently director of research in the Neag School of Education at the University of Connecticut as well as a professor in the department of kinesiology. Dr. Kraemer, a trained endocrinologist and neuromuscular physiologist, is a world-renowned expert in exercise physiology, sports medicine, and strength and conditioning. He is a fellow of the American College of Sports Medicine, chairs NASA's oversight committee on strength training for astronauts and cosmonauts at the International Space Station, and is editor in chief of the *Journal of Strength and Conditioning Research*. Previously, Dr. Kraemer worked at Pennsylvania State University, where he held multiple appointments, including director of research for the Center for Sports Medicine and associate director of the Center for Cell Research. In addition, Dr. Kraemer was the exercise physiology chair at Ball State University while heading the Human Performance Laboratory and serving as an adjunct professor of physiology and biophysics at the Indiana University School of Medicine. He advises ESPN sports network and many sports magazines on strength-training and fitness program content, he was a member of the U.S. Olympic Committee for Science and Technology and author of numerous scientific articles, books, and chapters, many of which focus on weight training, and he is always in demand as a lecturer.

David E. Krebs, Ph.D., PT, is a professor of physical therapy and clinical investigation at the Massachusetts General Hospital Institute of Health Professions, in Boston, Massachusetts, as well as the director of the Massachusetts General Hospital's Biomotion Laboratory. He also holds academic appointments in orthopedics at Harvard Medical School and mechanical engineering at the Massachusetts Institute of Technology. He was the twelfth annual Eugene Michels Researcher's Forum Featured Speaker of the American Physical Therapy Association and received its 1994 Golden Pen Award for Distinguished Scientific Writing.

Mario Lafortune, Ph.D., has directed the Nike Sports Research Laboratory since 1996. He received a doctoral degree in human biomechanics from Pennsylvania State University. Prior to joining Nike, Dr. Lafortune held positions at the University of Guelph in Canada and at the Australian Institute of Sports in Canberra, Australia. His research has focused on the understanding of the loads that act upon the human body during sporting activities. His work in that field earned him the award for the most significant contribution to footwear biomechanics at the Second International Symposium on Functional Footwear (1995). Dr. Lafortune has run several marathons and twice participated in the Hood to Coast 192-mile relay race in Oregon where he lives. Dr. Lafortune stays active by running between twenty and thirty miles per week and playing golf when the Oregon weather turns nice.

Mickey Levinson, PT, is clinical supervisor of the Sports Medicine Rehabilitation Department at the Hospital for Special Surgery in New York City. He was also the team physical therapist for the New York Mets baseball club from 1993 to 2000.

Gregory Lutz, M.D., is the chief of physiatry and the director of the Medical Spine Clinic at the Hospital for Special Surgery in New York City, as well as an associate professor of rehabilitation medicine at Weill Medical College of Cornell University.

Nancy Major, M.D., is an assistant professor at Duke University Medical Center, where she is on staff as a musculoskeletal radiologist with an appointment to orthopedic surgery. She did radiology residency training at the University of California at San Francisco and a musculoskeletal fellowship at Duke University. She is also a member of the International Skeletal Society and the Society of Skeletal Radiology in the Department of Radiology/Department of Surgery Division of Orthopaedics at Duke University.

Kathleen Mangione, Ph.D., PT, GCS, is an associate professor of physical therapy at Arcadia University in Glenside, Pennsylvania. She holds a B.S. in physical therapy from the University of Delaware, an M.A. in gerontology from New York University, and a Ph.D. in physical therapy from NYU. Dr. Mangione is very active in the American Physical Therapy Association (APTA), serving on the advisory board for research. She is also an associate editor for *Physical Therapy*.

Charles Matcan is a yoga instructor at the Manhattan Health Center.

Tim McAlindon, M.D., M.P.H., M.R.C.P., is an associate professor of medicine at the Boston University School of Medicine Arthritis Center. In addition, Dr. McAlindon is the director of the Internet Clinical Research Center at Boston University, where the focus is on "the development and validation of clinical research methodologies as applied over the Internet." He is a practicing rheumatologist at Boston Medical Center and holds positions in the Clinical Epidemiology Research and Training Unit and the Arthritis Center. His research interests include the epidemiology of rheumatic diseases such as osteoarthritis and the application of clinical research methodologies over the Internet.

Marian A. Minor, Ph.D., PT, is an associate professor in physical therapy, School of Health Professions, University of Missouri. Dr. Minor teaches in and leads a research program studying the benefits of exercise for people with arthritis. She received the Arthritis Foundation Engalitcheff Impact on Quality of Life Award in 2001 and is the 2001–2002 president of the Association of Rheumatology Health Professionals, a division of the American College of Rheumatology.

Howard Nelson, PT, has a B.S. in physical therapy and has worked in the physical therapy field for thirteen years. Formerly of the Hospital for Special Surgery, he is now working in private practice in New York City, specializing in orthopedics.

Michael C. Nevitt, Ph.D., is professor of epidemiology and biostatistics at the University of California at San Francisco. His research focuses on the epidemiology of and risk factors for osteoarthritis and osteoporosis.

David Nieman, Ph.D., is a professor of health and exercise science and the director of the Human Performance Lab at Appalachian State University in Boone, North Carolina.

Benno Nigg, Ph.D., is the director of the Human Performance Laboratory at the University of Calgary. Dr. Nigg is one of the world's foremost biomechanics researchers. His research includes the design of sports shoes and floor surfaces, improving the gait of amputee children, and measuring stress on the skeleton, tendons, ligaments, and other tissues. Dr. Nigg is regarded as the world's leading researcher on sports shoe construction.

Patrick J. Nunan, D.P.M., is a podiatrist in West Chester, Ohio, and president of the American Academy of Podiatric Sports Medicine. Dr. Nunan is also a fellow of the American Academy of Podiatric Sports Medicine, the American College of Foot and Ankle Orthopedics and Medicine, and the American College of Foot and Ankle Surgeons. Dr. Nunan is also the team podiatrist for Wilmington College in Ohio.

Judy Piette is a physical therapist at Georgia South Hand Therapy in Stockbridge, Georgia. She is on the medical advisory board for *Arthritis Today Magazine* as well as the medical and scientific committee for the Georgia Chapter of the Arthritis Foundation.

Fabian Pollo, Ph.D., earned his doctorate in biomedical engineering from Texas A&M University and is fellowship-trained in orthopedic biomechanics at the Hospital for Special Surgery in New York City. Dr. Pollo is director of research for the orthopedic surgery department at Baylor University Medical Center in Dallas and an adjunct faculty member in the Joint Biomedical Engineering Program at the University of Texas at Arlington and the University of Texas Southwestern Medical School.

David Z. Prince, M.D., FACP, is the director of cardiac rehabilitation at Montefiore Medical Center, New York City. In addition, Dr. Prince is an assistant professor of internal medicine and rehabilitation at the Albert Einstein College of Medicine.

Eric L. Radin, M.D., is semiretired and currently an adjunct professor of orthopedic surgery at the Tufts University School of Medicine. He has served on the medical faculties at Harvard, West Virginia University, and the University of Michigan. Dr. Radin studied medicine at Harvard and mechanical engineering at MIT and Oxford. He has been heavily involved in research on joints and the causes of osteoarthrosis since 1966.

Mark F. Reinking, a physical therapist and certified athletic trainer, is an assistant professor in the Department of Physical Therapy at Saint Louis University. Reinking is a board-certified specialist in sports physical therapy as recognized by the American Board of Physical Therapy Specialties. He has a bachelor's degree from Southwest Missouri State University, a master of science degree from Ohio State University, and a master of science degree from the University of Indianapolis. In addition to his teaching duties, Reinking provides physical therapy and athletic training clinical services for the athletic department at SLU.

Cheryl Riegger-Krugh, Sc.D., is a physical therapist and assistant professor at the University of Colorado Health Sciences Center. Dr. Riegger-Krugh's research interests include movement strategies and functional outcomes for people with hip and knee osteoarthrosis and lower-limb skeletal malalignment. In her clinical practice, Dr. Riegger-Krugh specializes in lower-limb skeletal malalignments and lower-limb osteoarthrosis. Dr. Riegger-Krugh has worked with Dr. Eric Radin on several osteoarthrosis studies.

Jeffrey A. Ross, D.P.M., is a fellow of the American College of Foot and Ankle Surgeons and the American College of Sports Medicine. Dr. Ross is also the former president of the American Academy of Podiatric Sports Medicine and an assistant clinical professor at Baylor College of Medicine. In addition, Dr. Ross is the cochair of the Governor's Fitness Council in Texas, a marathoner, a triathlete, and a columnist for *Inside Texas Running* magazine.

Neil S. Roth, M.D., is an assistant professor of orthopedic surgery specializing in sports medicine, shoulder, knee, and elbow surgery at the Columbia-Presbyterian Medical Center in New York City.

Leena Sharma, M.D., is an assistant professor at Northwestern University. Dr. Sharma's research focuses on identifying the determinants of structural disease progression and functional status decline in knee osteoarthritis. Recently, Dr. Sharma and her colleagues completed a one-of-a-kind study demonstrating knee alignment as a factor in the progression of knee osteoarthritis.

Kevin Sims is a private practitioner and clinical researcher in the physiotherapy department at the University of Queensland, Australia.

Stephen J. Sontag, M.D., is a staff physician at the Hines Veterans Administration Hospital in Hines, Illinois. Dr. Sontag is the developer of an important concept in this book, stiff man syndrome. Dr. Sontag has done much work in this area. He received his medical degree from the Chicago Medical School. After a one-year internship at Mount Sinai Hospital in Chicago, he moved to the Veterans Administration Hospital in Hines, Illinois, and remained for two years of residency training in internal medicine and two years of fellowship training in gastroenterology. Since 1977, Dr. Sontag has been a staff physician at Hines in the Medical Departments of Ambulatory Care and Gastroenterology. In his first five years at Hines, he also served as assistant professor of clinical medicine at the University of Illinois Abraham Lincoln School of Medicine. For the next twenty years he served on the staff at Loyola University Stritch School of Medicine, where he is currently a professor of medicine.

Tim Stump, M.S., PT, CSCS, is a licensed physical therapist and NSCA-certified strength and conditioning specialist. He has nine years of clinical experience in orthopedics and sports medicine and extensive experience working with high-level athletes at the college, professional, and Olympic level.

Anthony R. Temple, M.D., is vice president of medical and regulatory science for the McNeil Consumer & Specialty Pharmaceuticals Division of McNeil-PPC, Inc., North America's leading producer of over-the-counter pharmaceuticals. Dr. Temple, a pediatrician and clinical pharmacologist/medical toxicologist, has been involved in research and review of over-the-counter analgesics for more than thirty years. Dr. Temple is an adjunct associate professor, Department of Pediatrics, at the University of Pennsylvania School of Medicine.

Claudia L. Thomas, M.D., is assistant professor of orthopedic surgery in the Department of Orthopaedics at Johns Hopkins University School of Medicine. She is a graduate of the Johns Hopkins School of Medicine and the Yale orthopedic residency program. Dr. Thomas is board certified in orthopedic surgery and is a fellow of the American

Academy of Orthopaedic Surgeons. She is the first African-American female orthopedic surgeon in the United States.

Richard Ulin, M.D., is a clinical professor of orthopedics at the Mount Sinai Hospital in New York City. His specialty is orthopedic surgery, and his interests include elbow surgery, hand surgery, hip surgery, kyphosis/scoliosis, and spondylolysthesis.

Vijay B. Vad, M.D., is a physiatrist at the Hospital for Special Surgery in New York City. In addition, Dr. Vad is an assistant professor of rehabilitation medicine at Cornell University Medical Center. Dr. Vad is a consulting physician of the Professional Golfers' Association tour and Association of Tennis Professionals circuit in New York City.

Vassilios Vardaxis, Ph.D., is a clinical biomechanist and assistant professor of biomechanics/gait analysis at Indiana University. Dr. Vardaxis's research focuses on the understanding and identification of the mechanical characteristics of normal and pathological locomotion. Currently he is focusing on the identification of adult gait patterns that may lead to knee osteoarthritis predisposition due to mechanical loading.

Kevin E. Wilk, PT, a world-renowned physical therapist, is currently the national director of research and clinical education for HealthSouth Rehabilitation Corporation in Birmingham, Alabama. Wilk is also the associate clinical director of the HealthSouth Sports Medicine and Rehabilitation Center and director of rehabilitative research for the American Sports Medicine Institute. In addition, he is the rehabilitation consultant for the Tampa Bay Devil Rays baseball team. Wilk has published more than ninety-five journal articles and seventy-five book chapters and has lectured internationally and nationally at more than four hundred professional and scientific meetings. He is a clinician, researcher, and educator and is considered one of the leading therapists in cases of shoulder, knee, and elbow joint injury.

BIBLIOGRAPHY

Alaranta, H., H. Hurri, M. Heliovaara, A. Soukka, and R. Harju. "Non-dynamic Trunk Performance Tests: Reliability and Normative Data." *Scandinavian Journal of Rehabilitation Medicine* 26 (1994): 211–215.

Altman, R. D., M. C. Hochberg, R. W. Moskowitz, and T. J. Schnitzer. "Recommendations for the Medical Management of Osteoarthritis of the Hip and Knee." *Arthritis & Rheumatism* 43, no. 9 (2000): 1905–1915.

American Podiatric Medical Association. "APMA Frequently Asked Questions." www.apma.org/faqgeneral.html (February 2001).

Aviad, A. D., and J. B. Houpt. "The Molecular Weight of Therapeutic Hyaluronan (Sodium Hyaluronate): How Significant Is It?" *Journal of Rheumatology* 21 (1994): 297–301.

Berman, B. M., B. B. Singh, L. Lao, P. Langenberg, H. Li, V. Hadhazy, J. Bareta, and M. Hochberg. "A Randomized Trial of Acupuncture as an Adjunctive Therapy in Osteoarthritis of the Knee." *Rheumatology* 38, no. 4 (1999): 346–354.

Bombardier, C., L. Laine, A. Reicin, D. Shapiro, R. Burgos-Vargas, B. Davis, R. Day, M. B. Ferraz, C. J. Hawkey, M. C. Hochberg, T. K. Kvien, and T. J. Schnitzer (VIGOR Study Group). "Comparison of Upper Gastrointestinal Toxicity of Rofecoxib and Naproxen in Patients with Rheumatoid Arthritis." *New England Journal of Medicine* 343, no. 21 (2000): 1520–1528, plus 2 pp. following 1528.

Brand, C., J. Snaddon, M. Bailey, and F. Cicuttini. "Vitamin E Is Ineffective for Symptomatic Relief of Knee Osteoarthritis: A Six Month Double Blind, Randomised, Placebo Controlled Study." *Annals of Rheumatic Diseases* 60, no. 10 (2001): 946–949.

Brandt, K. D. "Putting Some Muscle into Osteoarthritis." *Annals of Internal Medicine* 127 (1997), 138–141.

Brandt, K. D., editor. *Rheumatic Disease Clinics of North America,* vol. 24, no. 25 (Philadelphia: W. B. Saunders, 1999).

Corle, D. K., C. Sharbaugh, D. J. Mateski, T. Coyne, E. D. Paskett, J. Cahill, C. Daston, E. Lanza, and A. Schatzkin. "Self-Rated Quality of Life Measures: Effect of Change to a Low-Fat, High-Fiber, Fruit and Vegetable Enriched Diet." *Annals of Behavioral Medicine* 23, no. 3 (2001): 198–207.

Deyle, G. D., N. E. Henderson, R. L. Matekel, M. G. Ryder, M. B. Garber, and S. C. Allison. "Effectiveness of Manual Physical Therapy and Exercise in Osteoarthritis of the Knee." *Annals of Internal Medicine* 132, no. 3 (2000): 173–181.

Dougados, M., M. Nguyen, L. Berdah, B. Mazieres, E. Vignon, and M. Lequesne (ECHODIAH Investigators Study Group). "Evaluation of the Structure-Modifying Effects of Diacerein in Hip Osteoarthritis: ECHODIAH, a Three-Year, Placebo-Controlled Trial. Evaluation of the Chondromodulating Effect of Diacerein in OA of the Hip." *Arthritis & Rheumatism* 44, no. 11 (2001): 2539–2547.

Eckhoff, D. G., W. K. Montgomery, R. F. Kilcoyne, and F. R. Stamm. "Femoral Morphometry and Anterior Knee Pain." *Clinical Orthopaedics* 302 (1994): 64–68.

Escamilla, R. F. "Knee Biomechanics of the Dynamic Squat Exercise." *Medicine and Science in Sports and Exercise* 33 (2001): 127–141.

Escamilla, R. F., G. S. Fleisig, N. Zheng, S. W. Barrentine, K. E. Wilk, and J. R. Andrews. "Biomechanics of the Knee During Closed Kinetic Chain and Open Kinetic Chain Exercises." *Medicine and Science in Sports and Exercise* 30, no. 4 (1998): 556–569.

Escamilla, R. F., G. S. Fleisig, N. Zheng, J. E. Lander, S. W. Barrentine, J. R. Andrews, B. W. Bergemann, and C. T. Moorman 3rd. "Effects of Technique Variations on Knee Biomechanics During the Squat and Leg Press." *Medicine and Science in Sports and Exercise* 33, no. 9 (2001): 1552–1566.

Ettinger, W. H., Jr., R. Burns, S. P. Messier, W. Applegate, W. J. Rejeski, T. Morgan, S. Shumaker, M. J. Berry, M. O'Toole, J. Monu, and T. Craven. "A Randomized Trial Comparing Aerobic Exercise and Resistance Exercise with a Health Education Program in Older Adults with Knee Osteoarthritis. The Fitness Arthritis and Seniors Trial (FAST)." *Journal of the American Medical Association* 277, no. 1 (1997): 25–31.

Felson, D. T. "The Epidemiology of Knee Osteoarthritis: Results from the

Framingham Osteoarthritis Study." *Seminars in Arthritis Rheumatology* 20 (1990): 42–50.

Felson, D. T., R. C. Lawrence, M. C. Hochberg, T. McAlindon, P. A. Dieppe, M. A. Minor, S. N. Blair, B. M. Berman, J. F. Fries, M. Weinberger, K. R. Lorig, J. J. Jacobs, and V. Goldberg. "Osteoarthritis: New Insights. Part 2: Treatment Approaches." *Annals of Internal Medicine* 133, no. 9 (2000): 726–737.

Garfinkel, M., and H. R. Schumacher, Jr. "Yoga." *Rheumatic Disease Clinics of North America* 26, no. 1 (2000): 125–132.

Garfinkel, M., H. R. Schumacher, Jr., A. Husain, M. Levy, and R. A. Reshetar. "Evaluation of a Yoga Based Regimen for Treatment of Osteoarthritis of the Hands." *Journal of Rheumatology* 21, no. 12 (1994): 2341–2343.

Gelber, A. C., M. C. Hochberg, L. A. Mead, N. Y. Wang, F. M. Wigley, and M. J. Klag. "Joint Injury in Young Adults and Risk for Subsequent Knee and Hip Osteoarthritis." *Annals of Internal Medicine* 133, no. 5 (2000): 321–328.

Hurley, M. V. "Quadriceps Weakness in Osteoarthritis." *Current Opinion in Rheumatology* 10 (1998): 246–250.

Hurley, M. V., and D. L. Scott. "Improvements in Quadriceps Sensorimotor Function and Disability of Patients with Knee Osteoarthritis Following a Clinically Practicable Exercise Regime." *British Journal of Rheumatology* 37 (1998): 1181–1187.

Hurley, M. V., D. L. Scott, J. Rees, and D. J. Newham. "Sensorimotor Changes and Functional Performance in Patients with Knee Osteoarthritis." *Annals of Rheumatic Diseases* 56 (1997): 641–648.

Keeler, L. K., L. H. Finkelstein, W. Miller, and B. Fernhall. "Early-Phase Adaptations of Traditional-Speed vs. Superslow Resistance Training on Strength and Aerobic Capacity in Sedentary Individuals." *Journal of Strength and Conditioning Research* 15, no. 3 (2001): 309–314.

Kerrigan, D. C., J. L. Lelas, and M. E. Karvosky. "Women's Shoes and Knee Osteoarthritis." *The Lancet* 357, no. 9262 (2001): 1097–1098.

Kerrigan, D. C., P. O. Riley, T. J. Nieto, and U. Della Croce. "Knee Joint Torques: A Comparison Between Women and Men During Barefoot Walking." *Archives of Physical Medicine and Rehabilitation* 81, no. 9 (2000): 1162–1165.

Kettunen, J. A., U. M. Kujala, J. Kaprio, M. Koskenvuo, and S. Sarna. "Lower-Limb Function Among Former Elite Male Athletes." *American Journal of Sports Medicine* 29, no. 1 (2001): 2–8.

Kirwan, J. R., and E. Rankin. "Intra-Articular Therapy in Osteoarthritis." *Baillieres Clinical Rheumatology* 11 (1997): 769–794.

Lane, N. E., L. R. Gore, S. R. Cumming, M. C. Hochberg, J. C. Scott, E. N. Williams, and M. C. Nevitt. "Serum Vitamin D Levels and Incident Changes of Radiographic Hip Osteoarthritis: A Longitudinal Study. Study of Osteoporotic Fractures Research Group." *Arthritis & Rheumatism* 42, no. 5 (1999): 854–860.

Lee, E.-O., R. Song, S.-C. Bae Seoul, and C. An. "Effects of a 12 Week Tai Chi Exercise Program on Pain, Balance, Muscle Strength, and Physical Functioning in Older Patients with Osteoarthritis: Randomized Trial." Abstract no. 20431 at the American College of Rheumatology Annual Scientific Meeting, San Francisco, November 2001.

Maheu, E., B. Mazieres, J. P. Valat, G. Loyau, X. Le Loet, P. Bourgeois, J. M. Grouin, and S. Rozenberg. "Symptomatic Efficacy of Avocado/Soybean Unsaponifiables in the Treatment of Osteoarthritis of the Knee and Hip: A Prospective, Randomized, Double-Blind, Placebo-Controlled, Multicenter Clinical Trial with a Six-Month Treatment Period and a Two-Month Followup Demonstrating a Persistent Effect." *Arthritis & Rheumatism* 41, no. 1 (1998): 81–91.

Mangione, K. K., K. McCully, A. Gloviak, I. Lefebvre, V. Hofmann, and R. Craik. "The Effects of High Intensity and Low Intensity Cycle Ergometry in Older Adults with Knee Osteoarthritis." *Journals of Gerontology: Medical Sciences* 54A (1999): M184–M190.

McAlindon, T. E., P. Jacques, Y. Zhang, M. T. Hannan, P. Aliabadi, B. Weissman, D. Rush, D. Levy, and D. T. Felson. "Do Antioxidant Micronutrients Protect Against the Development and Progression of Knee Osteoarthritis?" *Arthritis & Rheumatism* 39, no. 4 (1996): 648–656.

McAlindon, T. E., M. P. LaValley, J. P. Gulin, and D. T. Felson. "Glucosamine and Chondroitin for Treatment of Osteoarthritis: A Systematic Quality Assessment and Meta-analysis." *Journal of the American Medical Association* 283, no. 11 (2000): 1469–1475.

Messier, S. P., R. F. Loeser, M. N. Mitchell, G. Valle, T. P. Morgan, W. J. Rejeski, and W. H. Ettinger. "Exercise and Weight Loss in Obese Older Adults with Knee Osteoarthritis: A Preliminary Study." *Journal of the American Geriatric Society* 48, no. 9 (2000): 1062–1072.

Micheli, L. J. "Self-Test for Muscle Imbalance." *Georgia Tech Sports Medicine & Performance Newsletter* 10 (2001): 3.

Minor, M. A. "Exercise in the Management of Osteoarthritis of the Knee and Hip." *Arthritis Care and Research* 7, no. 4 (1994): 198–204.

Minor, M. A., and J. E. Hewett. "Physical Fitness and Work Capacity in Women with Rheumatoid Arthritis." *Arthritis Care and Research* 8, no. 3 (1995): 146–154.

Nevitt, M. C. "Chinese in Beijing Have a Very Low Prevalence of Hip OA Compared to U.S. Caucasians." Paper presented at the meeting of the American College of Rheumatology, Philadelphia, Pa., October 2000.

Orecchio, A. B. "Rehabilitation: Effectiveness Questions Confound Experts." *BioMechanics Magazine Knee Supplement* (2000).

Orien, W. P. "Equipment: Treadmill Use Alters Gait Mechanics." *BioMechanics Magazine* 7 (2000): 59–70.

Pelletier, J. P., D. Lajeunesse, P. Reboul, F. Mineau, J. C. Fernandes, P. Sabouret, and J. Martel-Pelletier. "Diacerein Reduces the Excess Synthesis of Bone Remodeling Factors by Human Osteoblast Cells from Osteoarthritic Subchondral Bone." *Journal of Rheumatology* 28, no. 4 (2001): 814–824.

Radin, E. L., K. H. Yang, C. Riegger, V. L. Kish, and J. J. O'Connor. "Relationship Between Lower Limb Dynamics and Knee Joint Pain." *Journal of Orthopaedic Research* 9, no. 3 (1991): 398–405.

Raynor, H. A., and L. H. Epstein. "Dietary Variety, Energy Regulation, and Obesity." *Psychological Bulletin* 127, no. 3 (2001): 325–341.

Reginster, J. Y., R. Deroisy, L. C. Rovati, R. L. Lee, E. Lejeune, O. Bruyere, G. Giacovelli, Y. Henrotin, J. E. Dacre, and C. Gossett. "Long-Term Effects of Glucosamine Sulphate on Osteoarthritis Progression: A Randomised, Placebo-Controlled Clinical Trial." *The Lancet* 357, no. 9252 (2001): 251–256.

Rogind, H., B. Bibow-Nielsen, B. Jensen, H. C. Moller, H. Frimodt-Moller, and H. Bliddal. "The Effects of a Physical Training Program on Patients with Osteoarthritis of the Knees." *Archives of Physical Medicine and Rehabilitation* 79, no. 11 (1998): 1421–1427.

Rolls, B. J., P. M. van Duijvenvoorde, and E. T. Rolls. "Pleasantness Changes and Food Intake in a Varied Four-Course Meal." *Appetite* 5, no. 4 (1984): 337–348.

Sadovsky, R. "Physical Therapy and Exercise for Osteoarthritis of the Knee." *American Family Physician* 61, no. 12 (2000): 3727.

Sadowski, T., and J. Steinmeyer. "Effects of Non-steroidal Antiinflammatory Drugs and Dexamethasone on the Activity and Expression of Matrix Metalloproteinase-1, Matrix Metalloproteinase-3 and Tissue

Inhibitor of Metalloproteinases-1 by Bovine Articular Chondrocytes." *Osteoarthritis & Cartilage* 9, no. 5 (2001): 407–415.

Sandmark, H. "Musculoskeletal Dysfunction in Physical Education Teachers." *Occupation and Environmental Medicine* 57, no. 10 (2000): 673–677.

Scheiman, J. M. "Preventing NSAID Toxicity to the Upper Gastrointestinal Tract." *Current Treatment Options in Gastroenterology* 2, no. 3 (1999), 205–213.

Schiodt, F. V., F. A. Rochling, D. L. Casey, and W. M. Lee. "Acetaminophen Toxicity in an Urban County Hospital." *New England Journal of Medicine* 337, no. 16 (1997): 1112–1117.

Sharma, L., C. Lou, S. Cahue, and D. D. Dunlop. "The Mechanism of the Effect of Obesity in Knee Osteoarthritis: The Mediating Role of Malalignment." *Arthritis & Rheumatism* 43, no. 3 (2000): 568–575.

Sharma, L., J. Song, D. T. Felson, S. Cahue, E. Shamiyeh, and D. D. Dunlop. "The Role of Knee Alignment in Disease Progression and Functional Decline in Knee Osteoarthritis." *Journal of the American Medical Association* 286, no. 2 (2001): 188–195.

Skinner, H. B., and J. E. Scherger. "Identifying Structural Hip and Knee Problems: Patient Age, History, and Limited Examination May Be All That's Needed." *Postgraduate Medicine* 106, no. 7 (1999): 51–52, 55–56, 61–64.

Slemenda, C., D. K. Heilman, K. D. Brandt, B. P. Katz, S. A. Mazzuca, E. M. Braunstein, and D. Byrd. "Reduced Quadriceps Strength Relative to Body Weight: A Risk Factor for Knee Osteoarthritis in Women?" *Arthritis & Rheumatism* 41, no. 11 (1998): 1951–1959.

Sontag, S. J., and J. N. Wanner. "The Cause of Leg Cramps and Knee Pains: An Hypothesis and Effective Treatment." *Medical Hypothesis* 25, no. 1 (1998): 35–41.

Steinkamp, L. A., M. F. Dillingham, M. D. Markel, J. A. Hill, and K. R. Kaufman. "Biomechanical Considerations in Patellofemoral Joint Rehabilitation." *American Journal of Sports Medicine* 21, no. 3 (1993), 438–444.

Stuart, M. J., D. A. Meglan, G. E. Lutz, E. S. Growney, and K.N. An. "Comparison of Intersegmental Tibiofemoral Joint Forces and Muscle Activity During Various Closed Kinetic Chain Exercises." *American Journal of Sports Medicine* 24, no. 6 (1996): 792–799.

Sun, W. Y. "Impact of Tai Chi Chuan Program on the Health Among Older Adults." *Student Monographs* 12, no. 1 (1994): 73–80.

Wernicke, G., and R. S. Panush. "Running and the Musculoskeletal System." *Bulletin on the Rheumatic Diseases* 50, no. 11 (2001): 1–3.

Wolfe, M. M., D. R. Lichtenstein, and G. Singh. "Gastrointestinal Toxicity of Nonsteroidal Antiinflammatory Drugs." *New England Journal of Medicine* 340, no. 24 (1999): 1888–1899.

Zhang, Y., L. Xu, M. C. Nevitt, P. Aliabadi, W. Yu, M. Qin, L. Y. Lui, and D. T. Felson. "Comparison of the Prevalence of Knee Osteoarthritis Between the Elderly Chinese Population in Beijing and Whites in the United States: The Beijing Osteoarthritis Study." *Arthritis & Rheumatism* 44, no. 9 (2001): 2065–2071.

INDEX

ABOUT THE AUTHOR

DR. BOB ARNOT is one of the most recognized names in the medical and health professions. Formerly medical correspondent for the CBS Evening News and chief medical correspondent for *Today* and *Dateline* broadcasts, Dr. Arnot now reports worldwide from the front lines of the war against terror as special foreign correspondent for MSNBC.

A bestselling author, Dr. Arnot has published eight books: *Sports Selection, The Best Medicine, Dr. Bob Arnot's Guide to Turning Back the Clock, Dr. Bob Arnot's Revolutionary Weight Control Program, The Breast Cancer Prevention Diet, The Biology of Success, The Prostate Cancer Protection Plan,* and *The Breast Health Cookbook.*